HPNA PALLIATIVE NURSING MANUALS

Physical Aspects
of Care

HPNA PALLIATIVE NURSING MANUALS

Series edited by: Betty R. Ferrell, RN, PhD, MA, FAAN, FPCN, CHPN

Volume 1: Structure and Processes of Care

Volume 2: Physical Aspects of Care: Pain and Gastrointestinal Symptoms

Volume 3: Physical Aspects of Care: Nutritional, Dermatologic, Neurologic and Other Symptoms

Volume 4: Pediatric Palliative Care

Volume 5: Social Aspects of Care

Volume 6: Spiritual, Religious, and Existential Aspects of Care and Cultural Aspects

Volume 7: Care of the Patient at the End of Life

Volume 8: Ethical and Legal Aspects

HPNA PALLIATIVE NURSING MANUALS

Physical Aspects of Care: Pain and Gastrointestinal Symptoms

Edited by

Judith A. Paice, PhD, RN, FAAN

Director of Cancer Pain Program
Division of Hematology-Oncology
Feinberg School of Medicine
Northwestern University Chicago, Illinois

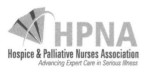

Hospice & Palliative Nurses Association
Advancing Expert Care in Serious Illness

OXFORD
UNIVERSITY PRESS

OXFORD

UNIVERSITY PRESS

Oxford University Press is a department of the University of
Oxford. It furthers the University's objective of excellence in research,
scholarship, and education by publishing worldwide.

Oxford   New York
Auckland   Cape Town   Dar es Salaam   Hong Kong   Karachi
Kuala Lumpur   Madrid   Melbourne   Mexico City   Nairobi
New Delhi   Shanghai   Taipei   Toronto

With offices in
Argentina   Austria   Brazil   Chile   Czech Republic   France   Greece
Guatemala   Hungary   Italy   Japan   Poland   Portugal   Singapore
South Korea   Switzerland   Thailand   Turkey   Ukraine   Vietnam

Oxford is a registered trademark of Oxford University Press
in the UK and certain other countries

Published in the United States of America by
Oxford University Press
198 Madison Avenue, New York, NY 10016

© Oxford University Press 2015

Library of Congress Cataloging-in-Publication Data
Physical aspects of care: pain and gastrointestinal symptoms / edited by Judith A. Paice.
p.; cm.—(HPNA palliative nursing manuals)
"Content for this series was derived primarily from the Oxford Textbook of Palliative Nursing
(4th edition, 2015), edited by Betty R. Ferrell, Nessa Coyle, Judith A. Paice. The Textbook
contains more extensive content and references so users of these Palliative Nursing Manuals are
encouraged to use the Textbook as an additional resource."—Preface.
Includes bibliographical references and index.
ISBN 978–0–19–023944–2 (alk. paper)
I. Paice, Judith A., editor.   II. Hospice and Palliative Nurses Association.
III. Oxford textbook of palliative nursing. 4th edition. 2014. Based on (expression):
IV. Series: HPNA palliative nursing manuals; v. 2.
[DNLM: 1. Hospice and Palliative Care Nursing.   2. Palliative Care—methods.
3. Terminal Care—methods. WY 152.3]
R726.8
616.02′9—dc23
2014036632

9 8 7 6 5 4 3 2
Printed in the United States of America
on acid-free paper

Contents

Preface

This is the second volume of a new series being published by Oxford University Press in collaboration with the Hospice and Palliative Nurses Association. The intent of this series is to provide palliative care nurses with quick reference guides to each of the key domains of palliative care.

Content for this series was derived primarily from the *Oxford Textbook of Palliative Nursing* (4th edition, 2015), which is also edited by Betty Ferrell, Nessa Coyle, and Judith Paice, the editors of this series. The contributors identified in each volume are the authors of chapters in the *Oxford Textbook of Palliative Nursing* from which the content was selected for this volume. The Textbook contains more extensive content and references, so users of these Palliative Nursing Manuals are encouraged to use the Textbook as an additional resource.

We are grateful to all palliative care nurses who are contributing to the advancement of care for seriously ill patients and families. Remarkable progress has occurred over the past 30 years in this field, and nurses have been central to that progress. Our hope is that this series offers an additional tool to build the care delivery system we strive for.

Contributors

Denice Caraccia Economou, RN, MN, CHPN
Senior Research Specialist
City of Hope National
    Medical Center
Duarte, California

Kimberley Chow, NP-BC, RN
Department of Palliative Care &
    Pain Management
Memorial Sloan-Kettering
    Cancer Center
New York, New York

Daniel Cogan, GNP-BC, ACHPN
Director of Palliative Care
Nassau University Medical Center
East Meadow, New York

Constance Dahlin, ANP-BC, ACHPN, FPCN, FAAN
Clinical Director
Palliative Care Service
Massachusetts General Hospital
Boston, Massachusetts

Regina M. Fink, RN, PhD, AOCN, FAAN
Research Nurse Scientist
University of Colorado Hospital
Cordillera, Colorado

Rose A. Gates, RN, PhD, AOCN, NP
Adult Nurse Practitioner,
    Oncology
Rock Mountain Cancer Center
Colorado Springs, Colorado

Audrey Kurash Cohen, MS, CCC-SLP
Clinical Speech Language
Pathologist
Boston, Massachusetts

Robert K. Montgomery, RN, ND
Coordinator of Pain Service
University of Colorado Hospital
Cordillera, Colorado

Chapter 1

Pain Assessment

Regina M. Finka, Rose A. Gates, and Robert K. Montgomery

This chapter considers various types of pain, describes barriers to optimal pain assessment, and reviews current clinical practice guidelines for the assessment of pain in the palliative care setting. A multifactorial model for pain assessment is proposed, and a variety of instruments and methods that can be used to assess pain in nonverbal and cognitively impaired patients are reviewed.

Types of Pain

According to the International Association for the Study of Pain (IASP), pain is defined as "an unpleasant sensory or emotional experience associated with actual or potential tissue damage. The inability to communicate verbally does not negate the possibility that an individual is experiencing pain and is in need of appropriate pain-relieving treatment."[1] Pain has also been clinically defined as "whatever the experiencing person says it is, existing whenever the experiencing person says it does."[2]

Pain is commonly categorized along a continuum of duration.

- Acute pain may be associated with tissue damage, inflammation, a disease process that is relatively brief, or a surgical procedure. Regardless of its intensity, acute pain is usually of brief duration: hours, days, weeks, or a few months. Acute pain serves as a warning that something is wrong and is generally viewed as a time-limited experience.

- Persistent or chronic pain worsens and intensifies with the passage of time, lasts for an extended period (months, years, or a lifetime), and adversely affects the patient's functioning or well-being. In the literature, the words "persistent" and "chronic" have often been used interchangeably to describe long-lasting pain. This newer term "persistent" is favored as it avoids the negative stereotype often associated with the label "chronic pain patient."

Pain can also be classified along pathophysiological terms that can assist the healthcare professional to determine the cause of pain and select the appropriate pain management interventions. Four pain subcategories have been delineated:

- Nociceptive pain (visceral or somatic pain resulting from stimulation of pain receptors)

- Neuropathic pain (pain caused by peripheral or central nervous system stimulation)
- Mixed or unspecified pain (having mixed or unknown pain mechanisms)
- Pain due to psychological disorders

Barriers to Optimal Pain Assessment

Multiple barriers to the achievement of optimal pain assessment and management have been identified (Box 1.1).[3–7] The knowledge and attitudes of healthcare professionals toward pain assessment are extremely important, because these factors influence the priority placed on pain treatment.

Process of Pain Assessment

Accurate pain assessment is the basis of pain treatment; it is a continuous process that encompasses multidimensional factors. In formulating a pain management plan of care, an assessment is crucial to identify the pain syndrome or the cause of pain. A comprehensive assessment addresses each type of pain and includes the following:

- Detailed history, including an assessment of the pain intensity, its characteristics, and its effects on function
- History of previous substance abuse
- Physical examination with pertinent neurological examination, particularly if neuropathic pain is suspected. Include examination of the painful areas and of common referred pain locations. Physical examination maneuvers and diagnostic tests should be performed only if the findings will potentially change or facilitate the treatment plan.
- Psychosocial and cultural assessment
- Appropriate diagnostic workup to determine the cause of pain. Attention should be paid to any discrepancies between patients' verbal descriptions of pain and their behavior and appearance.

Patients or residents should be asked whether they have pain (screened for pain) on admission to a hospital, clinic, nursing home, hospice, or home care agency. If pain or discomfort is reported, a comprehensive pain assessment should be performed at regular intervals, whenever there is a change in the pain, and after any modifications in the pain management plan.

- Reassessment of pain intensity should occur after each pain management intervention, once a sufficient time has elapsed for the treatment to reach peak effect (e.g., 15–30 minutes after a parenteral medication and within 1 hour of oral medication administration or other nonpharmacological intervention).
- The frequency of pain assessment and reassessment is determined by the patient's or resident's clinical situation.
- Pain assessment and reassessment should be individualized and documented so that all multidisciplinary team members involved will have an understanding of the pain problem.

Box 1.1 Barriers to Optimal Pain Assessment[3-7]

Healthcare Professional Barriers

Lack of identification of pain assessment and relief as a priority in patient care

Inadequate knowledge about how to perform a pain assessment

Perceived lack of time to conduct and document a pain assessment and reassessment

Failure to use validated pain measurement tools

Inability of clinician to empathize or establish rapport with patient

Lack of continuity of care

Lack of communication among the healthcare professional team

Prejudice and bias in dealing with patients

Failure to accept patient's/resident's pain reports

Healthcare System Barriers

A system that fails to hold healthcare professionals accountable for pain assessment

Lack of criteria or availability of culturally sensitive instruments for pain assessment in healthcare settings

Lack of institutional policies for performance and documentation of pain assessment

Patient/Family/Societal Barriers

The highly subjective and personal nature of the pain experience

Lack of patient and family awareness about the importance of speaking out about pain

Lack of patient communication with healthcare professionals about pain

- Patient reluctance to report pain
- Patient not wanting to bother staff
- Patient fears of not being believed
- Patient age-related stoicism
- Patient doesn't report pain because "nothing helps"
- Pain presence is a sign of deterioration
- Patient concern that curative therapy might be curtailed with pain and palliative care
- Lack of a common language to describe pain
- Presence of unfounded beliefs and myths about pain and its treatment

Multifactorial Model for Pain Assessment

Pain is a complex phenomenon involving many interrelated factors. Given the complexity of the interactions among the factors, if a positive impact on the quality of life of patients is the goal of palliative care, then the multifactorial perspective provides the foundation for assessing and managing pain. Some questions that can guide a multifactorial pain assessment are reviewed in Table 1.1.

Physiological and Sensory Factors

The physiological and sensory factors of the pain experience explain the cause of and characterize the person's pain. Patients should be asked to describe their pain, including its quality, intensity, location, temporal pattern, and aggravating and alleviating factors.

Words

Patients are asked to describe their pain or discomfort using words or qualifiers (Table 1.2). Identifying the qualifiers enhances understanding of the patient's pain etiology and should optimize pain treatment.

Intensity

Although an assessment of intensity captures only one aspect of the pain experience, it is the most frequently used parameter in clinical practice. In using these tools, patients typically are asked to rate their pain on a scale of 0 to 10: no pain = 0; mild pain is indicated by a score of 1 to 3; moderate pain, 4 to 6; and severe pain, 7 to 10.[8] Pain intensity should be evaluated not only at the present level but also at its least, worst, and average level and at rest or with movement. Pain intensity can be measured quantitatively with the use of a variety of instruments (Table 1.3)[9–22]:

- Visual analog scale
- Numeric rating scale
- Verbal descriptor scale
- Faces scale
- Pain thermometer

Table 1.1 Multifactorial Pain Assessment

Factors	Question
Physiologic/ sensory	What is causing the patient's pain?
	How does the patient describe his/her pain?
Affective	How does the patient's emotional state affect his/her report of pain?
	How does pain influence the patient's affect or mood?
Cognitive	How do the patient's knowledge, attitudes, and beliefs affect their pain experience?
	What is the meaning of the pain to the patient?
	How does the patient's past experience with pain influence the pain?
Behavioral	How do you know the patient is in pain?
	What patient pain behaviors or nonverbal cues inform you that pain is being experienced?
	What is the patient doing to decrease his or her pain?
Sociocultural	How does the patient's sociocultural background affect the pain experience, expression, and coping?
Environmental	How does the patient's environment affect the pain experience or expression?

Table 1.2 Pain Descriptors

Pain Type	Qualifiers	Possible Etiological Factors	Intervention
Neuropathic	Numb, burning, radiating, shooting, electrical, tingling, "pins and needles"	Injury to peripheral or central nervous tissue Nerve involvement by tumor (cervical, brachial, lumbosacral plexuses), postherpetic or trigeminal neuralgia, diabetic neuropathies, HIV-associated neuropathy (viral or antiretrovirals), chemotherapy-induced neuropathy, post-stroke pain, post-radiation plexopathies, phantom pain	Anticonvulsants, antidepressants, local anesthetics, ±opioids (e.g., tramadol, methadone), ±steroids, nerve blocks
Visceral (poorly localized)	Crampy, gnawing, deep, squeezing, pressure, stretching, bloated	Bowel obstruction, venous occlusion, ischemia, liver metastases, ascites, thrombosis, post abdominal or post thoracic surgery, pancreatitis	Opioids (caution must be used in the administration of opioids to patients with bowel obstruction), nonsteroidal antiinflammatory drugs (NSAIDs)
Somatic (well localized)	Aching, dull, throbbing, sore	Activation or injury of nociceptors/pain fibers in superficial cutaneous and deep musculoskeletal structures Bone or spine metastases, fractures, arthritis, osteoporosis, immobility	NSAIDs, ± opioids, steroids, muscle relaxants, bisphosphonates, radiation therapy (bone metastasis)
Psychologic	All-encompassing, everywhere	Psychologic disorders	Psychiatric treatments, support, non-pharmacological approaches

Location

The majority of persons with cancer have pain in two or more sites; therefore, it is crucial to ask questions about pain location. Encourage the patient to point or place a finger on the area involved. This will provide more specific data than verbal self-report.

Duration

Learning whether the pain is constant, intermittent, or both will guide the selection of interventions. Patients may experience "breakthrough" pain (BTP), an intermittent, transitory flare of pain, with several subtypes described:

Table 1.3 Pain Intensity Assessment Scales

Scale	Description	Advantages	Disadvantages
Visual Analogue Scale (VAS)	A horizontal or vertical line of 10 cm (or 100 mm) in length anchored at each end by verbal descriptors (e.g., no pain and worst possible pain). Patients are asked to make a slash mark or X on the line at the place that represents the amount of pain experienced. Often used in research studies.	Positive correlation with other self-reported measures of pain intensity and observed pain behaviors. Qualities of ratio data with high number of response categories make it more sensitive to changes in pain intensity.	Scoring may be more time-consuming and involve more steps. Patients may have difficulty using and understanding a VAS measure. Too abstract for many adults, and may be difficult to use with elderly, non-English-speaking, and patients with physical disability, immobility, or reduced visual acuity, which may limit their ability to place a mark on the line.
Numeric Rating Scale (NRS)	The number that the patient gives represents his/her pain intensity from 0 to 10 with the understanding that 0 = no pain and 10 = worst pain possible.	May be used with most children over 8 years of age. Verbal administration to patients allows those by phone or who are physically and visually disabled to quantify pain intensity. Ease in scoring, high compliance, high number of response categories. Scores may be treated as interval data and are correlated with VAS.	Lack of research comparing sensitivity to treatments impacting pain intensity.
Verbal Descriptor Scale (VDS)	Adjectives reflecting extremes of pain are ranked in order of severity. Each adjective is given a number, which constitutes the patient's pain intensity.	Short, ease of administration to patients, easily comprehended, high compliance. Easy to score and analyze data on an ordinal level. Validity is established.	Patients must choose one word to describe their pain intensity even if no word accurately describes it. Variability in use of verbal descriptors may be associated with affective distress. Scores on VDS are considered ordinal data; however, the distances between its descriptors are not equal but categorical. Less reliable among illiterate patients and persons with limited English vocabulary.

(continued)

Table 1.3 (Continued)

Scale	Description	Advantages	Disadvantages
FACES Scale	The scale consists of six cartoon-type faces. The no pain (0) face shows a widely smiling face and the most pain (10) face shows a face with tears. The scale is treated as a Likert scale and was originally developed to measure children's pain intensity or amount of hurt. It has been used in adults.	Simplicity, ease of use, and correlation with VAS makes it a valuable option in clinical settings. Short, requires little mental energy and little explanation for use.	Presence of tears on the "most pain" face may introduce cultural bias when the scale is used by adults from cultures not sanctioning crying in response to pain.
FACES Pain Scale—Revised (FPS-R)	The FACES Pain Scale Revised (FPS-R) was adapted from the FPS (seven faces) in order to make it compatible with a 0–10 metric scale. The FPS-R measures pain intensity and consists of six oval faces ranging from a neutral face (no pain) to a grimacing, sad face without tears (worst pain).	Easy to administer. Oval-shaped faces without tears or wide smiles are more adult-like in appearance, possibly making the scale more acceptable to adults. Recommended for use in research studies on the basis of utility and psychometric features	Facial expressions may be difficult to discern for patients who have visual difficulties. The FPS-R may measure other constructs (anger, distress, and impact of pain on functional status) than just pain intensity.
Pain Thermometer	Modified vertical verbal descriptor scale that is administered by asking the patient to point to the words that best describe his/her pain.	Increased sensitivity. Preferred for patients with moderate to severe cognitive deficits or those with difficulty with abstract thinking and verbal communication.	Allow for practice time to use this tool.

- Incidental
- Spontaneous
- End-of-dose pain

Aggravating and Alleviating Factors

If the patient is not receiving satisfactory pain relief, inquiring about what makes the pain worse or better—the aggravating and alleviating factors—will assist in determining which diagnostic tests need to be ordered or which nonpharmacological approaches can be incorporated into the plan of care. Pain interference with functional status can be measured by determining the pain's effects on activities such as function (walking or repositioning in bed), energy, falling and/or staying asleep, relationships, mood, or appetite.

Affective Factor

The affective factor includes the emotional responses associated with the pain experience and, possibly, such reactions as depression, anger, distress, anxiety, decreased ability to concentrate, mood disturbance, and loss of control. A person's feelings of distress, loss of control, or lack of involvement in the plan of care may affect outcomes of pain intensity and patient satisfaction with pain management.

Cognitive Factor

The cognitive factor refers to the way pain influences the person's thought processes; the way the person views himself or herself in relation to the pain; the knowledge, attitudes, and beliefs the person has about the pain and its management; and the meaning of the pain to the individual. Past experiences with pain may influence one's beliefs about pain A comprehensive approach to pain assessment includes evaluation of the patient's knowledge and beliefs about pain and its management and common misconceptions about analgesia (Box 1.2).

Behavioral Factor

Pain behaviors may be a means of expressing or coping with pain. These may include:

- Verbal complaints
- Moaning or groaning
- Crying
- Facial expressions
- Posturing
- Splinting
- Lying down
- Pacing
- Rocking
- Guarding a body part
- Rubbing

Sociocultural Factor

The sociocultural factor encompasses all of the demographic variables of the patient experiencing pain. Ultimately, all of these factors can influence pain assessment.

- Age: Elderly patients suffer disproportionately from chronic painful conditions and have multiple diagnoses with complex problems and accompanying pain. Elders have physical, social, and psychological needs distinct from those of younger and middle-aged adults, and they present particular challenges for pain assessment and management.
- Gender: Gender differences affect sensitivity to pain, pain tolerance, pain distress, willingness to report pain, exaggeration of pain, and nonverbal expression of pain.
- Ethnicity: The term "ethnicity" can refer to one or more of the following: (1) a common language or tradition, (2) shared origins or social

> ### Box 1.2 Common Patient Concerns and Misconceptions About Pain and Analgesia[5,6]
>
> Pain is inevitable. I just need to bear it.
>
> If I tell about my pain it may lead to a loss of independence and more tests.
>
> If the pain is worse, it must means my disease (cancer) is spreading.
>
> I had better wait to take my pain medication until I really need it or else it won't work later.
>
> My family thinks I am getting too "spacey" on pain medication; I'd better hold back.
>
> If it's morphine, I must be getting close to the end.
>
> If I take pain medicine (such as opioids) regularly, I will get "hooked" or addicted.
>
> If I take my pain medication before I hurt, I will end up taking too much. It's better to "hang in there and tough it out."
>
> I'd rather have a good bowel movement than take pain medication and get constipated.
>
> I don't want to bother the nurse or doctor; they're busy with other patients.
>
> If I take too much pain medication, it will hasten my death.
>
> Admitting I have pain is a sign of weakness.
>
> Good patients avoid talking about pain.

background, and (3) shared culture and traditions that are passed through generations and create a sense of identity. Ethnicity may be a predictor of pain expression and response. While assessing pain, it is important to remember that certain ethnic groups and cultures have strong beliefs about expressing pain and may hesitate to complain of unrelieved pain.

- Marital Status and Social Support: The degree of family or social support in a patient's life should be assessed, because these factors may influence the expression, meaning, and perception of pain and the ability to comply with therapeutic recommendations.

- Spirituality: The spiritual dimension may influence the person's pain response, expression, and experience. Whereas pain refers to a physical sensation, suffering refers to the quest for meaning, purpose, and fulfillment. Unrelieved physical pain may cause emotional or spiritual suffering, yet suffering may occur in the absence of pain. Assessing a patient's existential view of pain, suffering, and spiritual pain is important because it can affect the processes of healing and dying.

- Environmental Factor: The environmental factor refers to the environment in which the person receives pain management. Creating a peaceful environment free from bright lights, extreme noise, and excessive heat or cold may assist in alleviating the patient's pain. Context of care, setting, or where the patient receives care may also refer to the environmental aspect.

Pain Assessment in Nonverbal or Cognitively Impaired Patients

Obtaining the patient's self-report, the gold standard for pain assessment, is not always feasible with patients who cannot verbalize their pain and patients with severe cognitive impairment (e.g., dementia and delirium). The inability to communicate effectively due to impaired cognition and sensory losses is a serious problem for many patients with life-threatening illness. Observation of behaviors or surrogate reporting must be used in persons who cannot verbally communicate their pain. Pain assessment can be guided by the following principles and framework:

1. Use the hierarchy of pain assessment techniques[23,24]
   a. Obtain self-report, if possible.
   b. Search for potential causes of pain or other pathologies that could cause pain.
   c. Observe patient behaviors that are indicative of pain.
   d. Obtain proxy reporting (family members, parents, caregivers) of pain and behavior/activity changes.
   e. Attempt an analgesic trial to assess a reduction in possible pain behaviors.
2. Establish a procedure for pain assessment.
3. Use behavioral pain assessment tools, as appropriate.
4. Minimize emphasis on physiologic indicators.
5. Reassess and document.

Pain Behaviors

It may be more complicated to assess nonverbal cues in the palliative care setting because seriously ill patients with persistent pain, in contrast to patients with acute pain, may not demonstrate any specific behaviors indicative of pain. It is also unreasonable and even inaccurate to assess pain by relying on involuntary physiological bodily reactions, such as increases in blood pressure, pulse, or respiratory rate and depth. Elevated vital signs may occur with sudden, severe pain, but they usually do not occur with persistent pain after the body reaches physiological equilibrium. Examples of pain behaviors in cognitively impaired or nonverbal patients or residents are displayed in Table 1.4. Box 1.3 includes important questions to consider when caring for nonverbal patients who may be in pain.

Instruments Used to Assess Pain in Nonverbal or Cognitively Impaired Patients

Pain Behavioral Scales

Assessing pain in patients/residents who are nonverbal or cognitively impaired and are unable to verbally self-report pain presents a particular challenge to clinicians. An instrument that could detect the presence of or a reduction in pain behaviors could facilitate effective pain

Table 1.4 Possible Pain Behaviors in Nonverbal and Cognitively Impaired Patients or Residents

Behavior Category	Possible Pain Behaviors
Facial expressions	Grimace, frown, wince, sad or frightened look, wrinkled forehead, furrowed brow, closed or tightened eyelids, rapid blinking, clenched teeth or jaw
Body movements	Restless, agitated, jittery, "can't seem to sit still," fidgeting, pacing, rocking, constant or intermittent shifting of position, withdrawing
Protective mechanisms	Bracing, guarding, rubbing or massaging a body part, splinting, clutching or holding onto side rails, bed, tray table, or affected area during movement
Verbalizations	Saying common phrases such as "help me," "leave me alone," "get away from me," "don't touch me," "ouch," cursing, verbally abusive, praying out loud
Vocalizations	Sighing, moaning, groaning, crying, whining, oohing, aahing, calling out, screaming, chanting, breathing heavily
Mental status changes	Confusion, disorientation, irritability, distress, depression
Changes in activity patterns, routines, or interpersonal interactions	Decreased appetite, sleep alterations, decreased social activity participation, change in ambulation, immobilization, aggressive, combative, resisting care

Adapted from American Medical Directors Association. Pain Management in the Long-Term Care Setting: Clinical Practice Guideline. Columbia, MD: AMDA; 2012; Herr K, Bjoro K, Decker S. Tools for assessment of pain in nonverbal older adults with dementia: a state of the science review. J Pain Symptom Manage. 2006;31:170–192.

management plans. However, because pain is not just a set of pain behaviors, the absence of certain behaviors does not necessarily mean that the patient is pain free. There is no one current tool based on nonverbal pain behaviors that can be recommended for general applicability in clinical practice and palliative care settings. A basic summary of instruments used to assess pain in nonverbal or cognitively impaired patients is found in Table 1.5.[21,25–55]

Implications for Treatment

Although pain assessment in the nonverbal or cognitively impaired patient or resident presents a challenge to clinicians, it should not pose a barrier to optimal pain management. If patients are no longer able to verbally communicate whether they are in pain or not, the best approach is to assume that their underlying disease is still painful and to continue pain interventions based on analgesic history. Nonverbal patients should be empirically treated for pain if there is preexisting pain or evidence that any individual in a similar condition would experience pain. Likewise, palliative measures should be considered in nonverbal patients with behavior changes potentially related to pain.

Box 1.3 Assessment and Treatment of Pain in the Nonverbal or Cognitively Impaired Patient or Resident

- Is there a reason for the patient to be experiencing pain? Review the patient's diagnoses.
- Was the patient previously treated for pain? If so, what regimen was effective (include pharmacological and nonpharmacological interventions)?
- How does the patient usually act when he/she is in pain? (Note: The nurse may need to ask family/significant others or other healthcare professionals.)
- What is the family's/significant other's interpretation of the patient's behavior? Do they think the patient is in pain? Why do they feel this way?
- Try to obtain feedback from the patient, for example, ask patient to nod head, squeeze hand, move eyes up or down, raise legs, or hold up fingers to signal presence of pain.
- If appropriate, offer writing materials or pain intensity charts that patient can use or point to.
- If there is a possible reason for or sign of acute pain, treat with analgesics or other pain-relief measures.
- If a pharmacological or nonpharmacological intervention results in modifying pain behavior, continue with treatment.
- If pain behavior persists, rule out potential causes of the behavior (delirium, side effect of treatment, symptom of disease process); try appropriate intervention for behavior cause.
- Explain interventions to patient and family/significant other.

Table 1.5 Pain Assessment Tools for the Cognitively Impaired or Nonverbal Patient or Resident

Tool	Goal	Dimensions/ Parameters	Comments
Abbey Pain Scale	Assess pain in late-stage demented patients in nursing homes.	Vocalization Facial expression Change in body language Behavioral change Physiological change Physical change	Based on previous research, this scale was developed for use with end-/late-stage dementia residents unable to express needs. Six behavioral indicators are scored with four grades of severity (0 = absent through 3 = severe) for a total possible score of 18.

(continued)

Table 1.5 (Continued)

Tool	Goal	Dimensions/ Parameters	Comments
Assessment of Discomfort in Dementia Protocol (ADD)	Improve the recognition and treatment of pain and discomfort in patients with dementia who cannot report their internal states, with the added goal of decreasing inappropriate use of psychotropic medication administration.	Facial expression Mood Body language Voice Behavior	Based on items from the Discomfort Scale for Dementia of the Alzheimer Type (DS–DAT), the ADD protocol includes more overt symptoms (physical aggression, crying, calling out, resisting care, and existing behaviors). Protocol implementation when basic care interventions failed to ameliorate behavioral symptoms resulted in significant decreases in discomfort, significant increases in the use of pharmacological and nonpharmacological comfort interventions, and improved behavioral symptoms.
Certified Nurse Assistant Pain Assessment Tool (CPAT)	Assessment of pain in patients with severe dementia by nursing assistants	Facial expression Behavior Mood Body language Activity level	Developed as a nursing assistant–administered instrument. Each of the five items is scored (0–1) for the presence or absence of pain and summed for a total score ranging from 0 to 5; higher scores require evaluation by nursing staff.
Checklist of Nonverbal Pain Indicators (CNPI)	Measure pain behaviors in cognitively impaired elders.	Nonverbal Vocalizations Facial Grimaces/ winces Bracing Rubbing Restlessness Verbalizations	Rates the absence or presence of six behaviors, at rest and on movement. A summed score of the number of nonverbal pain indicators observed at rest and on movement is calculated (total possible score 0–12).

(continued)

Table 1.5 (Continued)

Tool	Goal	Dimensions/ Parameters	Comments
Critical Care Pain Observation Tool (CPOT)	Assess pain in adult patients in critical care who are unable to self-report	Facial expression Body movements Compliance with the ventilator (intubated patients) or Vocalization (extubated patients) Muscle tension	Each of the four domains is scored on three behaviors from 0 to 2 for a total score ranging from 0 to 8. Presence of pain is suspected at scores above 2 or when the score increases by 2 or more.
Discomfort Behavior Scale (DBS)	Identify discomfort in persons with cognitive impairment in nursing homes	Facial expression Verbalizations/ vocalizations Body language Changes in activity patterns or routines Mental status changes Changes in interpersonal interactions	Does not necessarily differentiate those in pain, but identifies those with discomfort that may be due to pain or other sources. Intended to be used quarterly with information from the Minimum Data Set for nursing homes and must be computer scored.
Disability Distress Assessment Tool (DisDAT)	Observe and identify discomfort in people with severely limited communication due to cognitive impairment or physical illness	Facial signs Vocal sounds Habits and mannerisms Body posture Body observation	The rater selects from a series of identical adjectives for each of the five categories to describe patient expression in both content and distressed states. There are a total of 77 descriptors of content and distressed states between the five categories. The tool loosely incorporates all six American Geriatric Society indicators of pain and is designed to identify behavior change from a content base line.

(continued)

Table 1.5 (Continued)

Tool	Goal	Dimensions/ Parameters	Comments
Discomfort Scale for Dementia of the Alzheimer Type (DS–DAT)	Measure discomfort, defined as a negative state, in elders with advanced dementia who have decreased cognition and verbalization.	Noisy breathing Negative vocalizations Contented facial expression Sad facial expression Frightened facial expression Frown Relaxed body language Tense body language Fidgeting	The negative state could be pain, anguish, or suffering. Scoring is based on evaluation of frequency, intensity, and duration of the behaviors and may be cumbersome, requiring more training and education than is feasible or realistic for clinicians in hospital or long-term care settings. As the DS–DAT has been criticized for being too complex for routine nursing care, it has been revised.
Doloplus-2	Assess pain in nonverbal elders experiencing chronic, persistent pain.	Somatic reactions (five items) • Somatic complaints • Protective body postures at rest • Protection of sore areas • Expression • Sleep pattern Psychomotor reactions (two items) • Washing and/or dressing • Mobility • Psychosocial reactions (three items) • Communication • Social life • Behavioral problems	Each of the 10 items is given a score (0–3) representing increased severity and summed for a total score ranging from 0 to 30. A total score of 5 or above indicates pain.

(continued)

Table 1.5 (Continued)

Tool	Goal	Dimensions/ Parameters	Comments
Elderly Pain Caring Assessment 2 (EPCA-2)	Observe and rate the intensity of both persistent and acute pain in nonverbal communicating older adults.	Observations before caregiver intervention • Facial expression • Spontaneous posture adopted at rest • Movements of the patient out of bed and/or in bed • Interaction of all kinds with other people Observations during caregiver intervention • Anxious anticipation of caregiver intervention • Reactions during caregiver intervention • Reactions of the patient when painful parts of the body nursed • Complaints voiced in the course of caregiving	Each item is rated on a 5-point scale from 0 (no pain) to 4 (intense pain). The total score is the sum of corresponding scores in the two dimensions. EPCA-2 is hypothesized to measure pain intensity through doctors', nurses', and other caregivers' proxy ratings of the presence and qualitative intensity of identified pain behaviors.
FLACC FLACC-R	Measure pain severity in postoperative children. Has also been tested in critically ill, cognitively impaired adults.	Face Legs Activity Cry Consolability	Each of the five items is given a score (0–2) representing increased severity and summed for a total score ranging from 0 to 10. The FLACC-R can be used for all nonverbal, cognitively impaired children. Parent-identified specific descriptors and unique behaviors have been added to the FLACC to improve its reliability and validity.

(continued)

Table 1.5 (Continued)

Tool	Goal	Dimensions/ Parameters	Comments
Mobilization-Observation-Behavior-Intensity-Dementia Pain Scale-2 (MOBID-2)	Observe pain behaviors and infer pain intensity at rest and with standardized guided activity in patients with severe cognitive impairment (SCI).	Facial expressions Pain noises Defensive gestures	Patient is moved through standardized guided movements of joints in hands/arms, legs and trunk; with each activity, caregiver observes for presence and intensity of pain on an 11-point NRS; caregiver assigns an independent overall pain intensity rating on an 11-point NRS. Incorporates patient self-report or expression, observation, and proxy assessment.
Multidimensional Objective Pain Assessment Tool (MOPAT)	Assess acute pain in non-communicative patients in hospice.	Behavioral Indicators • Restless • Tense muscles • Frowning/Grimacing • Patient sounds Physiological Indicators • Blood pressure • Heart rate • Respirations • Diaphoresis	Based on previous research, this tool has a four-item behavioral dimension ranked on a 3-point scale with 0 being none and 3 severe, and a three-item physiologic dimension rated as "no change from usual" or "change from usual." Both dimensions are summed for a total score of pain severity.
Non-communicative Patient's Pain Assessment Instrument (NOPPAIN)	Assessment of pain behaviors in patients with dementia by nursing assistants.	Care conditions under which pain behaviors are observed • Bathing • Dressing • Transfers Presence/absence of pain behaviors • Pain words • Pain noises • Pain faces • Bracing • Rubbing • Restlessness	Developed as a nursing assistant–administered instrument. Pain is observed at rest and on movement while nursing assistants perform resident care. Pain behaviors are observed, and pain intensity is scored using a pain thermometer.

(continued)

Table 1.5 (Continued)

Tool	Goal	Dimensions/ Parameters	Comments
		Pain behavior intensity using 6-point Likert scale Pain thermometer for rating overall pain intensity	
Pain Assessment for the Dementing Elderly (PADE)	Assess pain behaviors in patients with advanced dementia.	Physical • Facial expression • Breathing pattern • Posture Global • Proxy pain intensity Functional • Dressing • Feeding oneself • Wheelchair to bed transfers	Twenty-four items (three domains) were developed after a literature review, interviews with nursing staff, and observations of residents in a dementia unit.
Pain Assessment Tool in Confused Older Adults (PATCOA)	Observe nonverbal cues to assess pain in acutely confused older adults.	Quivering Guarding Frowning Grimacing Clenching jaws Points to where it hurts Reluctance to move Vocalizations of moaning Sighing	An ordinal scale includes nine items of nonverbal pain cues rated as absent or present while the patient is at rest; higher scores indicate higher pain intensity.
Pain Assessment in Advanced Dementia (PAINAD)	Assess pain in patients with advanced dementia.	Breathing (independent of vocalization) Negative vocalization Facial expression Body language Consolability	Derived from the behaviors and categories of the FLACC, DS-DAT, and clinicians' pain descriptors of dementia. The intent is to simply measure pain using a 0–10 score (each item is scored as 0–2 and summed) in noncommunicative individuals.

(continued)

Tool	Goal	Dimensions/Parameters	Comments
Pain Assessment Behavioral Scale (PABS)	Assess pain in nonverbal, critically ill hospital inpatients.	Face Restlessness Muscle tone Vocalization Consolability	Each of the five items is given a score (0–2) representing increased severity and summed for a total score ranging from 0 to 10. The patient is observed at rest and with movement. Two scores are generated; the higher score is documented.
Pain Assessment Checklist for Seniors with Limited Ability to Communicate (PACSLAC)	Assess common and subtle behaviors in seniors with advanced dementia.	Facial expressions Activity and body movements Social/personality/mood indicators Physiological indicators/eating and sleeping/vocal behaviors	Can differentiate between pain and distress; scores were positively correlated with cognitive impairment level.
Pain Behaviors for Osteoarthritis Instrument for Cognitively Impaired Elders (PBOICIE)	Assess osteoarthritis (OA) pain in the knee or hip for severely cognitively impaired elders.	Distorted ambulation or gesture • Excessive stiffness • Shifting weight • Clutching or holding area • Rigid, tense body posture • Massaging affected area • Facial/nonaudible expressions of distress • Clenching teeth	A dichotomous scale (absent or present) with scores total ranging from 0 to 6 is used; if the presence of one behavior on the PBOICIE is observed then it is indicative of the presence of pain. Limitation in practice setting based on use only in population with a specific diagnosis of OA.
Pain Assessment in Non-communicative Elderly Persons PAINE	Assess pain in non-communicative elders.	Facial expressions Verbalizations Body movements Changes in activity/patterns Nurse-identified physical and vocal behaviors Visible pain cues	Twenty-two-item scale with a 6-point rating scale (1 = never to 7 = several times an hour) to measure frequency of occurrence of pain behaviors.

References

1. Merskey H, Bogduk N, eds. Classification of Chronic Pain, 2nd ed. International Association for the Study of Pain, Task Force on Taxonomy. Seattle, WA: IASP Press; 1994:209–214.

2. McCaffery M. Nursing Practice Theories Related to Cognition, Bodily Pain, and Man-Environment Interactions. Los Angeles, CA: UCLA Press; 1968:95.

3. Reynolds J, Drew D, Dunwoody C. American Society of Pain Management Nursing Position Statement: Pain Management at the End of Life. Pain Manage Nurs. 2013;14(3):172–175.

4. Goldberg GR, Morrison RS. Pain management in hospitalized cancer patients: a systematic review. J Clin Oncol. 2007;25:1792–1801.

5. Jones K, Fink R, Clark L, Hutt E, Vojir CP, Mellis BK. Nursing home resident barriers to effective pain management: why nursing home residents may not seek pain medication. J Am Med Dir Assoc. 2005;6:10–17.

6. Borneman T, Koczywas M, Sun V, et al. Effectiveness of a clinical intervention to eliminate barriers to pain and fatigue management in oncology. J Palliat Med. 2011;14(2):197–205.

7. Pasero C, McCaffery M. Pain Assessment and Pharmacologic Management. St. Louis, MO: Elsevier Mosby; 2011.

8. National Comprehensive Cancer Network (NCCN). Adult Cancer Pain: Clinical Practice Guidelines in Oncology, version 2. 2013. Available at http://www.nccn.org/professionals/physician_gls/f_guidelines.asp#pain. Accessed September 11, 2013.

9. Jensen M. The validity and reliability of pain measures in adults with cancer. J Pain. 2003;4:2–21.

10. Revill SI, Robinson JO, Rosen M, Hogg MIJ. The reliability of a linear analogue for evaluating pain. Anaesthesia. 1976;31:1191–1998.

11. Herr KA, Mobily PR. Comparison of selected pain assessment tools for use with the elderly. Appl Nurs Res. 1993;6:39–49.

12. von Baeyer CL, Spagrud LJ, McCormick JC, Choo E, Neville K, Connelly MA. Three new datasets supporting use of the Numerical Rating Scale (NRS-11) for children's self-reports of pain intensity. Pain. 2009;143(3):223–227.

13. Paice JA, Cohen FL. Validity of a verbally administered numeric rating scale to measure cancer pain intensity. Cancer Nurs. 1997;20:88–93.

14. Ferraz MB, Quaresma MR, Aquino LRL, Atra E, Tugwell P, Goldsmith CH. Reliability of pain scales in the assessment of literate and illiterate patients with rheumatoid arthritis. J Rheumatol. 1990;17:1022–1024.

15. Hockenberry MJ, Wilson D. Wong's Essentials of Pediatric Nursing, 8th ed. St. Louis: Mosby; 2009.

16. Stuppy DJ. The Faces Pain Scale: reliability and validity with mature adults. Appl Nurs Res. 1998;11:84–89.

17. Casas JM, Wagenheim BR, Banchero R, Mendoza-Romero J. Hispanic masculinity: myth or psychological schema meriting clinical consideration. Hisp J Behav Sci. 1994;16:315–331.

18. Hicks CL, von Baeyer CL, Spafford P, van Korlaar I, Goodenough B. The Faces Scale-Revised: toward a common metric in pediatric pain measurement. Pain. 2001;93:173–183.

19. International Association for the Study of Pain. Available at http://www.iasp-pain.org/Content/NavigationMenu/GeneralResourceLinks/FacesPainScaleRevised/default.htm. Accessed September 27, 2013.

20. Bieri D, Reeve R, Champion GD, Addicoat L, Ziegler JB. The Faces Pain Scale for the self-assessment of the severity of pain experienced by children: development, initial validation, and preliminary investigation for ratio scale properties. Pain. 1990;41:139–150.

21. Tomlinson D, von Baeyer CL, Stinson JN, Sung L. A systematic review of faces scales for the self-report of pain intensity in children. Pediatrics. 2010;126(5):e1168–e1198.

22. Herr KA, Garand L. Assessment and management of pain in older adults. Clin Geriat Med. 2001;17:457–478.

23. Herr K, Coyne PJ, McCaffery M, Manworren R, Merkel S. Pain assessment in the patient unable to self-report: position statement with clinical practice recommendations. Pain Manage Nurs. 2011;12:230–250.

24. Hadijistavropoulos T, Herr K, Turk DC, et al. An interdisciplinary expert consensus statement on assessment of pain in older persons. Clin J Pain. 2007; 23:S1–S43.

25. American Medical Directors Association. Pain Management in the Long-Term Care Setting: Clinical Practice Guideline. Columbia, MD: AMDA; 2012.

26. Herr K, Bjoro K, Decker S. Tools for assessment of pain in nonverbal older adults with dementia: a state of the science review. J Pain Symptom Manage. 2006;31:170–192.

27. Abbey J, Piller N, De Bellis A, et al. The Abbey Pain Scale: a 1-minute numerical indicator for people with end-stage dementia. Int J Palliat Nurs. 2004;10:6–13.

28. Kovach CR, Weissman D, Griffie J, Matson S, Muchka S. Assessment and treatment of discomfort for people with late stage dementia. J Pain Symptom Manage. 1999;18:412–419.

29. Kovach CR, Noonan PE, Griffie J, Muchka S, Weissman DE. The Assessment of Discomfort in Dementia Protocol. Pain Manage Nurs. 2002;3:16–27.

30. Hurley AC, Volicer BJ, Hanrahan PA, Houde S, Volicer L. Assessment of discomfort in advanced Alzheimer patients. Res Nurs Health. 1992;15:369–377.

31. Cervo FA, Bruckenthal P, Chen JJ, Bright-Long LE, Fields S, Zhang G, et al. Pain assessment in nursing home residents with dementia: psychometric properties and clinical utility of the CNA pain assessment tool (CPAT). J Am Med Dir Assoc. 2009;10:505–510.

32. Feldt KS. The Checklist of Nonverbal Pain Indicators (CNPI). Pain Manage Nurs. 2000;1:13–21.

33. Gelinas C, Fillion L, Puntillo KA. Item selection and content validity of the critical-care pain observation tool for nonverbal adults. J Adv Nurs. 2009;65:203–216.

34. Gelinas C. Nurses' evaluations of the feasibility and the clinical utility of the critical-care pain observation tool. Pain Manage Nurs. 2010;11:115–125.

35. Stevenson K, Brown R, Dahl J, Ward S, Brown M. The discomfort behavior scale: a measure of discomfort in the cognitively impaired based on the minimum data set 2.0. Res Nurs Health. 2006;29:576–587.

36. Regnard C, Reynolds J, Watson B, Matthews D, Gibson L, Clarke C. Understanding distress in people with severe communication difficulties: developing and assessing the Disability Distress Assessment Tool (DisDAT). J Intellect Disability Res. 2007; 51: 277–292.

37. Warden V, Hurley AC, Volicer L. Development and psychometric evaluation of the Pain Assessment in Advanced Dementia (PAINAD) scale. J Am Med Dir Assoc. 2003;9–15.

38. Wary B. Doloplus-2: a scale for pain measurement. Soins Gerontol. 1999;19:25–27.

39. Pautex S, Herrmann F, Michon A, Giannakopoulos P, Gold G. Psychometric properties of the doloplus-2 observational pain scale and comparison to self-assessment in hospitalized elderly. Clin J Pain. 2007;23:774–779.

40. Morello R, Jean A, Alix M, et al. A scale to measure pain in non-verbally communicating older patients: the EPCA-2 study of its psychometric properties. Pain. 2007;133:87–98.

41. Merkel SI, Voepel-Lewis T, Shayevitz JR, Malviya S. The FLACC: a behavioral scale for scoring postoperative pain in young children. Pediatr Nurs. 1997;23:293–297.

42. Malviya S, Voepel-Lewis T, Burke C, Merkel S, Tait AR. The revised FLACC observational pain tool: improved reliability and validity for pain assessment in children with cognitive impairment. Paediatr Anaesth. 2006;16(3):258–265.

43. Voepel-Lewis T, Zanotti J, Dammeyer JA. Reliability and validity of the faces, legs, activity, cry, consolability behavioral tool in assessing acute pain in critically ill patients. Am J Crit Care. 2010;19(1):55–62.

44. Husebo BS, Strand LI, Moe-Nilssen R, Husebo SB, Ljunggren AE. Pain in older persons with severe dementia: psychometric properties of the Mobilization-Observation-Behaviour-Intensity-Dementia (MOBID2) Pain Scale in a clinical setting. Scan J Caring Sci. 2010;24(2):380–391.

45. McGuire DB, Reifsnyder J, Soeken K, Kaiser KS, Yeager KA. Assessing pain in nonresponsive hospice patients: development and preliminary testing of the multidimensional objective pain assessment tool (MOPAT). J Palliat Med. 2011;14:287–292.

46. Snow AL, Weber JB, O'Malley KJ, et al. NOPPAIN: a nursing assistant-administered pain assessment instrument for use in dementia. Dement Geriatr Cogn Disord. 2004;17:240–246.

47. Villanueva MR, Smith TL, Erickson JS, Lee AC, Singer C. Pain Assessment for the Dementing Elderly (PADE): reliability and validity of a new measure. J Am Med Dir Assoc. 2003;4:1–8.

48. Cohen-Manfield J, Lipson S. The utility of pain assessment for analgesic use in persons with dementia. Pain. 2008;134:16–23.

49. Decker SA, Perry AG. The development and testing of the PATCOA to assess pain in confused older adults. Pain Manage Nurs. 2003;4:77–86.

50. DeWaters T, Faut-Callahan M, McCann JJ, et al. Comparison of self-reported pain and the PAINAD scale in hospitalized cognitively impaired and intact older adults after hip fracture surgery. Orthop Nurs. 2008;27:21–28.

51. Campbell M. Psychometric Testing of a New Pain Assessment Behavior Scale (PABS). Abstract presented at the 29th Annual MNRS Research Conference, 2005.

52. Fuchs-Lacelle S, Hadjistavropoulos T. Development and preliminary validation of the Pain Assessment Checklist for Seniors with Limited Ability to Communicate (PACSLAC). Pain Manage Nurs. 2004;5:37–49.

53. Tsai PF, Beck C, Richards KC, et al. The pain behaviors for osteoarthritis instrument for cognitively impaired elders (PBOICIE). Res Gerontol Nurs. 2008;1:116–122.

54. Cohen-Mansfield J. Pain assessment in noncommunicative elderly persons—PAINE. Clin J Pain. 2006;22:569–575.

55. Cohen-Mansfield J, Lipson S. The utility of pain assessment for analgesic use in persons with dementia. Pain. 2008;134:16–23.

Chapter 2

Pain Management

Judith A. Paice

Pain is highly prevalent in palliative care, yet the majority of individuals can obtain good relief with available treatment options. These therapies include pharmacological agents, such as nonopioids, opioids, coanalgesics, cancer therapies, and, in some cases, interventional techniques. Nurses are critical members of the palliative care team, particularly in providing pain management. The nurse's role begins with assessment and continues through the development of a plan of care and its implementation. During this process, the nurse provides education and counsel to the patient, family, and other team members. Nurses also are critical for developing institutional policies and monitoring outcomes that ensure good pain management for all patients within their palliative care program. The Institute of Medicine's report *Relieving Pain in America* identified that effective pain control and alleviation of suffering results not from the clinician's intervention alone, but rather the strength of the clinician, patient, and family relationship.[1] This is a key strength of nursing at all phases of palliative care.

Prevalence of Pain

The prevalence of pain in the terminally ill varies by diagnosis and other factors.

- Cancer: Approximately one-third of persons who are actively receiving treatment for cancer and two-thirds of those with advanced malignant disease experience pain. Individuals at particular risk for undertreatment include the elderly, minorities, and women. Almost three-quarters of patients with advanced cancer admitted to the hospital experience pain at admission. Pain often is the dominant symptom in patients admitted to palliative care units, along with fatigue and dyspnea. Children dying of cancer also are at risk for pain and suffering.
- HIV: The prevalence of pain in those with human immunodeficiency virus (HIV) disease varies widely and can have a profound negative effect on quality of life. Headache, abdominal pain, chest pain, and neuropathies are the most frequently reported types of pain. Lower CD4 cell counts and HIV-1 RNA levels are associated with higher rates of neuropathy. Numerous studies have reported undertreatment of persons with HIV disease, including those patients with a history of addictive disease.

- Other disorders: Unfortunately, there has been little characterization of the pain prevalence and experience of patients with other life-threatening disorders. However, those working in palliative care are well aware that pain frequently accompanies many of the neuromuscular and cardiovascular disorders, such as multiple sclerosis and stroke, seen at the end of life. Furthermore, many patients in hospice and palliative care are elderly and more likely to have existing chronic pain syndromes, such as osteoarthritis or low back pain.

Effects of Unrelieved Pain

Although many professionals and laypersons fear that opioid analgesics lead to shortened life, there is significant evidence to the contrary.[2]

- A large cohort study revealed that individuals experiencing chronic pain had a 10-year increased mortality.[3]
- It is likely that inadequate pain relief hastens death by increasing physiological stress, potentially diminishing immunocompetence, decreasing mobility, worsening proclivities toward pneumonia and thromboembolism, and increasing work of breathing and myocardial oxygen requirements.

Therefore, it is the professional and ethical responsibility of clinicians to focus on, and attend to, adequate pain relief for their patients and to properly educate patients and their caregivers about all analgesic therapies.

Pharmacological Management of Pain in Advanced and End-Stage Disease

Pharmacological management of pain includes nonopioids, opioids, and coanalgesics.[4,5] Cancer therapies and, in some cases, interventional techniques may also be used in this care. A sound understanding of pharmacotherapy in the treatment of pain is of great importance in palliative care nursing, allowing the nurse to:

- Contribute to the comprehensive plan of care
- Recognize and assess medication-related adverse effects
- Understand drug–drug and drug–disease interactions
- Educate patients and caregivers regarding appropriate medication usage

Patients or family members are not always aware of the names of their medications, or they may bring pills to the hospital or clinic that are not in their original bottles. Several web-based resources provide pictures that can assist in identifying the current analgesic regimen (Box 2.1).

Nonopioid Analgesics

Acetaminophen

Acetaminophen is especially useful in the management of nonspecific musculoskeletal pains or pain associated with osteoarthritis, but acetaminophen (also abbreviated as APAP and referred to as paracetamol in the rest

Box 2.1 Pill Identification Resources
http://www.drugs.com/pill_identification.html http://pillbox.nlm.nih.gov/pillimage/search.php http://www.rxlist.com/pill-identification-tool/article.htm http://www.webmd.com/pill-identification/default.htm

of the world) should be considered an adjunct to any chronic pain regimen. Some considerations:

- Acetaminophen has limited antiinflammatory effects.
- Reduce doses or avoid acetaminophen when a patient has renal insufficiency or liver dysfunction.
- For patients with normal hepatic and renal function, maximum daily doses of 2000–3000 mg are recommended.
- Overdose can occur as patients/providers may not consider combined dosing of prescribed and over-the-counter (OTC) medications.
- An intravenous formulation of acetaminophen is currently available, although cost issues may limit its use in palliative care.

Nonsteroidal Antiinflammatory Drugs
Nonsteroidal antiinflammatory drugs (NSAIDs) affect analgesia by:

- Reducing the biosynthesis of prostaglandins, thereby inhibiting the cascade of inflammatory events that cause, amplify, or maintain nociception.
- Reduce pain by influences on the peripheral or central nervous system independent of their antiinflammatory mechanism of action. This secondary mode of analgesic efficacy is poorly understood.

The NSAIDs are very useful in the treatment of many pain conditions mediated by inflammation, including those caused by cancer. They may be useful for moderate to severe pain control, either alone or as an adjunct to opioid analgesic therapy. Relative contraindications include:

- Decreased renal function
- Hepatic dysfunction failure
- Platelet dysfunction or other bleeding disorders

Adverse effects include:

- Gastrointestinal ulceration
- Renal dysfunction
- Impaired platelet aggregation
- Cardiovascular risk, including myocardial infarction and stroke, appears to be higher in those with preexisting risk factors
  See Table 2.1 for acetaminophen and selected NSAID dosages.

Opioid Analgesics

As a pharmacological class, the opioid analgesics represent the most useful agents for the treatment of pain associated with advanced disease. The opioids are nonspecific insofar as they decrease pain signal transmission and

Table 2.1 Acetaminophen and Selected Nonsteroidal Antiinflammatory Drugs

Drug	Dose if Patient > 50 kg	Dose if Patient < 50 kg
Acetaminophen[*†]	500–1000 mg q 4–6h oral; maximum 2000–3000 mg/24 h 1000 mg q 6h IV (given over 15 minute infusion); maximum 4000 mg/24 h	10–15 mg/kg q 4h (oral) 15 mg/kg q 6h; maximum 75 mg (IV) 15–20 mg/kg q 4h (rectal)
Aspirin[*†]	4000 mg/24h maximum, given q 4–6h	10–15 mg/kg q 4h (oral) 15–20 mg/kg q 4h (rectal)
Ibuprofen[*†]	2400 mg/24h maximum, given q 6–8h	10 mg/kg q 6–8h (oral)
Naproxen[*†]	1000 mg/24h maximum, given q 8–12h	5 mg/kg q 8h (oral/rectal)
Choline magnesium trisalicylate[*§]	2000–3000 mg/24h maximum, given q 8–12 h	25 mg/kg q 8h (oral)
Indomethacin[†]	75–150 mg/24h maximum, given q 8–12h	0.5–1 mg/kg q 8–12h (oral/rectal)
Ketorolac[‡]	30–60 mg IM/IV initially, then 15–30 mg q 6h bolus IV/IM or continuous IV/SQ infusion; short-term use only (3–5 days)	0.25–1 mg/kg q 6h short-term use only (3–5 days)
Celecoxib[§¶]	100–200 mg PO up to BID.	No data available

[*] Commercially available in a liquid form.

[†] Commercially available in a suppository form.

[‡] Potent antiinflammatory (short-term use only due to gastrointestinal side effects).

[§] Minimal platelet dysfunction.

[¶] Cyclooxygenase-2-selective nonsteroidal antiinflammatory drug.

perception throughout the nervous system, regardless of the pathophysiology of the pain. Indications for the use of opioids include:

- Moderate to severe pain—the main clinical indication for the opioid analgesics
- Nociceptive and neuropathic pain, although higher doses may be warranted for neuropathic pain
- Treatment of dyspnea
- Use as an anesthetic adjunct during invasive procedures
- Treatment of psychological dependence to opioids (e.g., methadone maintenance for those with a history of heroin abuse)

Because misunderstandings lead to undertreatment, it is incumbent on all clinicians involved in the care of patients with chronic pain to clearly understand and differentiate the clinical conditions of tolerance, physical dependence, addiction, pseudoaddiction, and pseudotolerance (Box 2.2).

Box 2.2 Definitions of Patient Relationships With Opioid Analgesics

Addiction[5]

Addiction is a primary, chronic, neurobiological disease, with genetic, psychosocial, and environmental factors influencing its development and manifestations. It is characterized by behaviors that include one or more of the following: impaired control over drug use, compulsive use, continued use despite harm, and craving.

Physical Dependence

Physical dependence is a state of adaptation that is manifested by a drug-class-specific withdrawal syndrome that can be produced by abrupt cessation, rapid dose reduction, decreasing blood level of the drug, and/or administration of an antagonist.

Tolerance

Tolerance is a state of adaptation in which exposure to a drug induces changes that result in a diminution of one or more of the drug's effects overtime.

Pseudoaddiction

Pseudoaddiction is the mistaken assumption of addiction in a patient who is seeking relief from pain.

Pseudotolerance

Pseudotolerance is the misconception that the need for increasing doses of drug is due to tolerance rather than disease progression or other factors.

Guidelines for Opioid Use

There is significant inter- and intraindividual variation in clinical responses to the various opioids, so in most cases a dose-titration approach should be viewed as the best means of optimizing care.[6] This implies that close follow-up is required to determine when clinical endpoints have been reached. Furthermore, idiosyncratic responses may require trials of different agents to determine the most effective drug and route of delivery for any given patient. Box 2.3 lists more specific suggestions regarding optimal use of opioids.

Morphine

Morphine is most often considered the "gold standard" of opioid analgesics and is used as a measure for dose equivalence. Common early adverse effects (these can occur with all opioids) include:

- Itching
- Headache
- Dysphoria or euphoria
- Sedation

Box 2.3 Guidelines for the Use of Opioids[4,5]

Clinical studies and experience suggest that adherence to some basic precepts will help optimize care of patients who require opioid analgesic therapy for pain control:

- Oral administration of opioids is preferred in most cases. Intramuscular administration is highly discouraged. Subcutaneous or intravenous delivery is almost always an alternative.
- Noninvasive drug delivery systems that "bypass" the enteral route (e.g., the transdermal and the oral transmucosal routes for delivery of fentanyl for treatment of continuous pain and breakthrough pain, respectively) may obviate the necessity to use parenteral routes for pain control in some patients who cannot take medications orally or rectally.
- Anticipation, prevention, and treatment of sedation, constipation, nausea, psychotomimetic effects, and myoclonus should be part of every care plan for patients being treated with opioid analgesics.
- Changing from one opioid to another or from one route to another is often necessary, so facility with this process is an absolute necessity. Remember the following points:
  —Incomplete cross-tolerance occurs, leading to decreased requirements of a newly prescribed opioid.
  —Use morphine equivalents as a "common denominator" for all dose conversions in order to avoid errors.

- Nausea
- Constipation—an adverse effect that persists

Adverse effects associated with longer-term use can include:

- Diaphoresis
- Hypogonadism
- Hyperalgesia
- Myoclonus—metabolites of morphine and hydromorphone, morphine-3-glucuronide (M3G) and hydromorphone-3-glucuronide (H3G), respectively, may contribute to myoclonus, seizures, and hyperalgesia (increasing pain), particularly when patients cannot clear these metabolites due to renal impairment. However, a small study of hospice patients showed increased levels of either M3G or H3G were not correlated with the presence of myoclonus.

If adverse effects exceed the analgesic benefit of the drug, convert to an equianalgesic dose of a different opioid (Table 2.2). Because cross-tolerance is incomplete, reduce the calculated dose by one-third to one-half and titrate upward based on the patient's pain intensity.

Clinical considerations regarding morphine when swallowing is compromised:

- The 24-hour, long-acting morphine capsule can be broken open and the "sprinkles" placed in applesauce or other soft food.

Table 2.2 Approximate Equianalgesic Doses of Commonly Used Opioid Analgesics*

Drug	Parenteral Route	Enteral Route
Morphine[†]	10 mg	30 mg
Codeine	130 mg	200 mg (not recommended)
Fentanyl[‡†††]	50–100 mcg	TIRF[‡]
Hydrocodone	Not available	30 mg
Hydromorphone[§]	1.5 mg	7.5 mg
Levorphanol[¶]	2 mg acute, 1 chronic	4 mg acute, 1 chronic
Methadone[¶]	See text	See text
Oxycodone[**]	Not available	20 mg
Oxymorphone	1 mg	10 mg
Tramadol	100 mg	120 mg

* Dose conversion should be closely monitored since incomplete cross-tolerance may occur. Interindividual variation in duration of analgesic effect is not uncommon, signaling the need to increase the dose or shorten the dose interval.

† Available in continuous- and sustained-release pills and capsules, formulated to last 12 or 24 hours. Also available in transdermal and TIRF, see package insert materials for dose recommendations. TIRF = transmucosal immediate release fentanyl.

§ Available as a continuous-release formulation lasting 24 hours.

¶ These drugs have long half-lives, so accumulation can occur; close monitoring during first few days of therapy is very important.

** Available in several continuous-release doses, formulated to last 12 hours.

†† Fentanyl 100-mcg patch ≈ 4 mg IV morphine/h.

Adapted from Paice JA, Ferrell B. The management of cancer pain. CA Cancer J Clin. 2011;61(3):157–182; American Pain Society. Principles of Analgesic Use in the Treatment of Acute Pain and Cancer Pain. 6th ed. Glenview: American Pain Society; 2008.

- Oral morphine solution can be swallowed, or small volumes (0.5–1 mL) of a concentrated solution (e.g., 20 mg/mL) can be placed in the mouth of patients whose voluntary swallowing capabilities are more significantly limited.

- Transmucosal uptake of morphine is slow and unpredictable due to its hydrophilic chemical nature. In fact, most of the analgesic effect of a morphine tablet or liquid placed buccally or sublingually is due to drug trickling down the throat and the resultant absorption through the gastrointestinal tract.

- Due to the hydrophilic nature of morphine, creams, gels, and patches that contain morphine do not cross the skin and therefore do not provide systemic analgesia.[7]

- The rectal route, using commercially prepared suppositories, compounded suppositories, or microenemas, can be used to deliver the drug into the rectum or stoma. Sustained-release morphine tablets have been used rectally, with resultant delayed time to peak plasma level and approximately 90% of the bioavailability achieved by oral administration. However, consider whether family members can physically or culturally deliver the drug by this route.

Fentanyl

Fentanyl is a highly lipid soluble opioid that has been administered parenterally, spinally, transdermally, transmucosally (bucal, sublingual, and nasal) for pain control, and by nebulizer for the management of dyspnea. Because of its potency, dosing is usually conducted in micrograms.

Transdermal Fentanyl

Transdermal fentanyl, often called the fentanyl patch, is indicated:

- When patients cannot swallow.
- When patients or caregivers do not remember to take or administer medications.
- When patients have adverse effects to other opioids.

Possible indications, although additional research is needed:

- Intractable constipation—transdermal fentanyl may produce less constipation when compared with long-acting morphine.
- Pain relief associated with pancreatitis—At lower doses, transdermal fentanyl has limited effect on the sphincter of Oddi, suggesting that this may be a safe and effective therapy for patients with pancreatitis.

Two primary systems are currently available:

- A reservoir-based patch (i.e., Duragesic)—When exposed to heat there is greater drug permeation at 72 hours in the reservoir system.
- A matrix type patch (i.e., Mylan)—There is greater permeation of drug through the dermis of compromised skin when using the matrix patch.

Patients and families often require education regarding use of the patch (Box 2.4).

Factors that may influence use of transdermal fentanyl:

- Fever (may increase absorption of drug)
- Diaphoresis (can limit adherence of patch and alter absorption)
- Morbid obesity (thought to alter absorption and distribution of drug, although studies are lacking)
- Reduced hepatic function (altered metabolism)
- Concomitant use of CYP3A4 inducers (alter serum levels)
- Cachexia (one study found reduced serum levels, but this does not preclude use—may need to increase doses)

Some patients experience decreased analgesic effects after only 48 hours of applying a new patch; this should be accommodated by determining whether a higher dose is tolerated with increased duration of effect or a more frequent (q 48 h) patch change should be scheduled.

Transmucosal Immediate-Release Fentanyl Products

Several formulations of transmucosal immediate-release fentanyl (TIRF) products are available, including oral transmucosal fentanyl citrate

> **Box 2.4 Fentanyl Patch Instructions to Patients and Caregivers[4]**
>
> 1. Place patch on the upper body in a clean, dry, hairless area (clip hair, do not shave). The patch does not need to be placed over the site of pain.
> 2. Choose a different site when placing a new patch, then remove the old patch.
> 3. If a skin reaction consistently occurs despite site rotation, spray inhaled steroid (intended for inhalational use in asthma) over the area, let dry and apply patch (steroid creams prevent adherence of the patch).
> 4. Remove the old patch or patches and fold sticky surfaces together, and then flush down the toilet.
> 5. Wash hands after handling patches.
> 6. All unused patches (patient discontinued use or deceased) should be removed from wrappers, folded in half with sticky surfaces together, and flushed down the toilet.

(OTFC), buccal tablets, soluble film, and nasal spray.[8] Prescribers of these formulations must enroll in the TIRF-Risk Evaluation Mitigation Strategy.

- The OTFC is composed of fentanyl on an applicator that patients rub against the oral mucosa to provide rapid absorption of the drug. Patients should use OTFC over a period of 15 minutes because too-rapid use will result in more of the agent being swallowed rather than being absorbed transmucosally. Adults should start with the 200-mcg dose and monitor efficacy, advancing to higher dose units as needed. The around-the-clock dose of opioid does not predict the effective dose of OTFC.

- The fentanyl buccal tablet has been shown to be effective, and, when compared with OTFC, fentanyl buccal tablets produce a more rapid onset and greater extent of absorption. The adverse effects are similar to those seen with other opioids, although a small percentage of patients do not tolerate the sensation of the tablet effervescing in the buccal space. For patients who cannot place the tablet buccally (between the gum and cheek pouch), sublingual (under the tongue) administration produced comparable bioequivalence.

- Bioadhesive films impregnated with fentanyl are an alternate to tablet formulations, providing efficacy with few adverse effects.

- Fentanyl nasal spray has the most rapid onset of the TIRF products, with significantly improved pain intensity scores as early as 5 minutes after administration, along with minimal adverse effects.

Oxycodone

Oxycodone is a synthetic opioid available in a long-acting formulation (OxyContin), as well as immediate-release tablets (alone or with acetaminophen) and liquid.

- The equianalgesic ratio is approximately 20 mg oxycodone to 30 mg oral morphine.

- CYP3A4 may alter oxycodone pharmacokinetics; substances that inhibit CYP3A4, such as the highly active antiretroviral agent retonavir, the antiviral voriconazole, and even grapefruit juice, have been found to increase oxycodone concentrations. Lower doses of oxycodone may be warranted when CYP3A4 inhibitors are administered.

Methadone

Methadone has several characteristics that make it useful in the management of severe, chronic pain.[9]

- Long half-life of 24 to 60 hours or longer allows prolonged dosing intervals; for pain control, every-8-hour dosing is recommended.
- Methadone also binds as an antagonist to the N-methyl-D-aspartate (NMDA) receptor, believed to be of particular benefit in neuropathic pain.
- Methadone can be given orally, parenterally, and sublingually.
- Methadone is much less costly than comparable doses of continuous-release formulations.

However, several factors can make methadone challenging:

- The long half-life means upward dose titration should be performed very slowly, every 3–7 days, to avoid sedation and respiratory depression.
- Most recommend that methadone not be used for prn dosing, also due to long half-life.
- The dosing ratio between methadone and other opioids is not known, making rotation difficult.
- Methadone has been shown to lead to prolonged QTc wave changes (also called torsade de pointes).
- Serious drug-drug interactions can occur. Methadone is metabolized primarily by CYP3A4, but also by CYP2D6 and CYP1A2. As a result, drugs that induce CYP enzymes accelerate the metabolism of methadone, resulting in reduced serum levels of the drug. This may be demonstrated clinically by shortened analgesic periods or reduced overall pain relief. Drugs that inhibit CYP enzymes slow methadone metabolism, potentially leading to sedation and respiratory depression. Drugs commonly used in palliative care are listed in Table 2.3.

Close monitoring of these potentially adverse or even life-threatening effects is required, and most experts suggest that methadone only be prescribed by experienced clinicians.

Hydromorphone

Hydromorphone (Dilaudid) is a useful alternative when synthetic opioids provide an advantage. It is available in oral immediate release and long-acting tablets, liquids, suppositories, and a parenteral formulation.

- Although H3G may accumulate in renal disease, this metabolite is removed when patients are receiving dialysis.

Other Opioids

Buprenorphine, codeine, hydrocodone, levorphanol, oxymorphone, tramadol, and tapentadol are other opioids available in the United States for treatment of pain.

Table 2.3 Selected Medications That Increase or Decrease Methadone Serum Levels	
CYP3A4 Inducers That Decrease Methadone	**CYP3A4 Inhibitors That Increase Methadone**
Barbiturates	Cimetidine
Carbamazepine	Ciprofloxacin
Dexamethasone	Diazepam
Phenytoin	Haloperidol
Rifampin	Ketoconazole
Spironolactone	Omeprazole
	Verapamil

- Buprenorphine, a partial agonist, is available parenterally and as a 7-day patch approved for moderate to severe pain. It is also used as part of an opioid maintenance program instead of methadone.
- Codeine is limited by pharmacogenetics; as a prodrug it must be broken down by the enzyme CYP2D6 to provide analgesia, yet approximately 10% are poor metabolizers. Conversely, some patients are ultrarapid metabolizers, which can lead to overdose.
- Hydrocodone is available in combination products, limiting dose escalation in palliative care due to concerns regarding excess acetaminophen or other agents. More recently a long-acting product without acetaminophen or other agents has been approved.
- Levorphanol has similarities to methadone, including a longer half-life; it is difficult to obtain in the United States.
- Oxymorphone is a semisynthetic opioid that is available in oral immediate-release and extended-release tablets and a parenteral formulation.
- Tramadol is a weak opioid and has serotonin and norepinephrine reuptake inhibition properties. It is available in immediate- and extended-release formulations. Although tramadol is effective for neuropathic pain, a systematic review found insufficient data to recommend its use as an alternative to codeine for mild to moderate pain. Dose escalation is limited due to potential lowering of the seizure threshold.
- Tapentadol is available in immediate- and extended-release formulations, and initial reports suggest it may be useful in some palliative care settings.

Alternative Routes of Administration for Opioid Analgesics

Many routes of administration are available when patients can no longer swallow or when other dynamics preclude the oral route or favor other routes. These include:

- Parenteral (intravenous or subcutaneous)
- Transdermal
- Transmucosal
- Rectal/Enteral

- Topical
- Epidural or intrathecal

Parenteral administration includes subcutaneous and IV delivery (intramuscular opioid delivery is inappropriate in the palliative care setting).

- Subcutaneous boluses have a slower onset and lower peak effect when compared with IV boluses. Subcutaneous infusions may include up to 10 mL/h (although most patients absorb 2 to 3 mL/h with least difficulty). Volumes greater than 10 mL/h are poorly absorbed. Hyaluronidase has been reported to speed absorption of subcutaneously administered drugs.
- The IV route provides rapid drug delivery but requires vascular access, placing the patient at risk for infection and potentially complicating the care provided by family or other loved ones.
- Intraspinal routes, including epidural or intrathecal delivery, may allow administration of drugs, such as opioids, local anesthetics, and/or alpha-adrenergic agonists.
- May be useful when opioids given by other routes are poorly tolerated or ineffective.
- Limitations include complexity of delivery systems, requiring specialized knowledge for healthcare professionals and potentially greater caregiver burden, as well as increased cost.

Preventing and Treating Adverse Effects of Opioid Analgesics

Constipation

Patients in palliative care frequently experience constipation, in part due to opioid therapy.

- Always begin a prophylactic bowel regimen when commencing opioid analgesic therapy.
- Most clinicians recommend a laxative/softener combination, such as senna/docusate, although research is lacking.[10]
- Avoid bulking agents (e.g., psyllium), because these tend to cause a larger, bulkier stool, increasing desiccation time in the large bowel.
- Fluid intake should be encouraged whenever feasible, but alone is rarely sufficient.
- Methylnaltrexone, has been shown to be effective in relieving opioid-induced constipation when given subcutaneously at doses of 0.15 mg/kg.
- Lubiprostone, an oral agent that works on chloride channels in the intestine, was approved for use in opioid-induced constipation in noncancer patients.

Sedation

Excessive sedation may occur with the initial doses of opioids. If sedation persists after 24 to 48 hours and other correctable causes have been identified and treated, do the following if possible:

- Rotate the opioid.
- Consider the use of a psychostimulant such as dextroamphetamine 2.5 to 5 mg PO q morning and midday or methylphenidate 5 to 10 mg PO q morning and 2.5 to 5 mg midday (although higher doses are frequently used).

Respiratory Depression

Titration of opioid analgesics to effect pain relief in palliative care is rarely associated with induced respiratory depression and iatrogenic death. In a recent retrospective study of opioid use in a hospice setting, there was no relationship between opioid dose and survival. When respiratory depression occurs in a patient with advanced disease, the cause is usually multifactorial. Therefore, other factors beyond opioids need to be assessed, although opioids are frequently blamed for the reduced respirations. A relatively recently identified phenomenon is the onset, or exacerbation of, sleep apnea in patients taking opioids for pain. Although this has been described in nonmalignant pain populations, this may be of concern for some palliative care patients. Risk factors appear to include the following:

- Use of methadone
- Concomitant use of benzodiazepines or other sedative agents
- Respiratory infection
- Obesity (which is a risk factor for sleep apnea)

When undesired depressed consciousness occurs along with a respiratory rate less than 8/min or hypoxemia (O_2 saturation <90%) associated with opioid use, cautious and slow titration of naloxone, which reverses the effects of the opioids should be instituted.

- Dilute 1 ampule of naloxone (0.4 mg/mL) in 10 mL of injectable saline (final concentration 40 mcg/mL) and inject 1 mL every 2 to 3 minutes while closely monitoring the level of consciousness and respiratory rate.
- Excessive dosing or too rapid administration may cause abrupt opioid reversal with pain and autonomic crisis.
- Because the duration of effect of naloxone is approximately 30 minutes, the depressant effects of the opioid will recur at 30 minutes and persist until the plasma levels decline (often 4 or more hours) or until the next dose of naloxone is administered.

Nausea and Vomiting

Nausea and vomiting are common with opioids due to activation of the chemoreceptor trigger zone in the medulla, vestibular sensitivity, and delayed gastric emptying, but habituation occurs in most cases within several days.

- Assess for other treatable causes.
- Pharmacotherapy may include regular dosing of is indicated. The doses of nausea-relieving medications and antiemetics listed below are to be used initially but can be increased as required.

Myoclonus

Myoclonic jerking occurs more commonly with high-dose opioid therapy, although it has also been reported with lower dosing. If this should develop:

- Switch to an alternate opioid.
- Add a benzodiazepine, such as clonazepam 0.5 to 1 mg PO q 6 to 8 hours if the patient can swallow, lorazepam sublingually or parenterally if the patient is unable to swallow, or midazolam if parenteral dosing is needed.
- In some cases, an epidural or intrathecal approach can allow the delivery of other agents (local anesthetics, alpha-2 adrenergic

agents such as clonidine) to provide pain control and reduce opioid requirements.

Pruritus

Pruritus appears to be most common with morphine, in part due to histamine release, but can occur with most opioids. Fentanyl and oxymorphone may be less likely to cause histamine release.

- Antihistamines can be useful.
- Sedation is an adverse effect of diphenhydramine, consider nonsedating agents such as loratadine or cetirizine.
- Ondansetron has been reported to be effective in relieving opioid-induced pruritus, but no randomized controlled studies exist.
- Consider opioid rotation.

Coanalgesics

A wide variety of nonopioid medications from several pharmacological classes have been demonstrated to reduce pain caused by various pathological conditions (Table 2.4). Although they often reduce pain when used alone, in palliative care, when these drugs are indicated for the treatment of severe neuropathic pain or bone pain, opioid analgesics are used concomitantly to provide adequate pain relief.

Antidepressants

Both older antidepressants and newer atypical agents have been shown to be effective in relieving neuropathic pain, although there remains little support for the analgesic effect of serotonin selective reuptake inhibitors (SSRIs). Atypical antidepressants, venlafaxine and duloxetine, have been shown to reduce neuropathy associated with chemotherapy-induced neuropathy in experimental animal models and in humans. The delay in onset of pain relief, from days to weeks, may preclude the use of these agents for pain relief in end-of-life care. However, their sleep-enhancing and mood-elevating effects may be of benefit.

Anticonvulsants

The older anticonvulsants, such as carbamazepine and clonazepam, relieve pain by blocking sodium channels. Gabapentin and pregabalin act at the alpha-2 delta subunit of the voltage-gated calcium channel. Additional evidence supports the use of these agents in neuropathic pain syndromes seen in palliative care, such as thalamic pain, pain due to spinal cord injury, and cancer pain, along with restless leg syndrome. Pregabalin has undergone extensive testing in pain due to diabetic neuropathy and has been found to be effective. Withdrawal from either compound should be gradual.

Corticosteroids

Corticosteroids inhibit prostaglandin synthesis and reduce edema surrounding neural tissues. Dexamethasone has been found to reduce numerous symptoms:

- Postoperative pain and nausea after mastectomy
- Neuropathic syndromes, including plexopathies
- Right upper quadrant abdominal pain associated with stretching of the liver capsule due to metastases

Table 2.4 Adjuvant Analgesics

Drug Class	Daily Adult Starting Dose* (Range)	Routes of Administration	Adverse Effects	Indications
Antidepressants	Nortriptyline 10–25 mg	PO	Anticholinergic effects	Neuropathic pain
	Desipramine 10–25 mg	PO		
	Venlafaxine 37.5 mg BID	PO	Nausea, dizziness	
	Duloxetine 30 mg	PO	Nausea	
Anticonvulsants	Clonazepam 0.5–1 mg HS, BID, or TID	PO	Sedation	Neuropathic pain
	Carbamazepine 100 mg q day or TID	PO	Sedation, Aplastic anemia (rare)	
	Gabapentin 100 mg TID	PO	Sedation, dizziness	
	Pregabalin 50 mg BID or TID	PO	Sedation, dizziness	
Corticosteroids	Dexamethasone 2–20 mg q day; may give up to 100 mg IV bolus for pain crises	PO/IV/SQ	"Steroid psychosis," dyspepsia	Cerebral edema, spinal cord compression, bone pain, neuropathic pain, visceral pain
	Prednisone 15–30 mg TID	PO		
Local anesthetics	Mexiletine 150 mg TID	PO	Lightheadedness, arrhythmias	Neuropathic pain
	Lidocaine 1–5 mg/kg hourly	IV or SQ infusion		
N-Methyl-D-aspartate antagonists	Dextromethorphan, effective dose unknown	PO	Confusion	Neuropathic pain
	Ketamine	IV		

(continued)

Table 2.4 (Continued)

Drug Class	Daily Adult Starting Dose* (Range)	Routes of Administration	Adverse Effects	Indications
Bisphosphonates	Pamidronate 60–90 mg over 2h every 2–4 wk	IV infusion	Pain flare	Osteolytic bone pain
Calcitonin	25 IU/day	SQ/nasal	Hypersensitivity reaction, nausea	Neuropathic pain, bone pain
Capsaicin	0.025%–0.075%	Topical	Burning	Neuropathic pain
Baclofen	10 mg q day or TID	PO	Muscle weakness, cognitive changes	
Calcium channel blockers	Nifedipine 10 mg TID	PO	Bradycardia, hypotension	Ischemic pain, neuropathic pain, smooth muscle spasms with pain

* Pediatric doses for pain control not well established.

Adapted from Paice JA, Ferrell B. The management of cancer pain. CA Cancer J Clin. 2011;61(3):157–182; American Pain Society. Principles of Analgesic Use in the Treatment of Acute Pain and Cancer Pain. 6th ed. Glenview: American Pain Society; 2008.

- Referred pain
- Bone pain
- Malignant intestinal obstruction
- Fatigue due to its activating effect
- Anorexia (short term effect—2–3 weeks)

Dexamethasone produces the least amount of mineralocorticoid effect, leading to reduced potential for Cushing's syndrome. Recommendations:

- Available in oral, IV, subcutaneous, and epidural formulations
- Standard dose is 2 to 24 mg/day.
- Can be administered once daily due to the long half-life of this drug
- Doses as high as 100 mg may be given with severe pain crises
- Intravenous bolus doses should be pushed slowly, to prevent uncomfortable perineal burning and itching.

Local Anesthetics

Local anesthetics work in a manner similar to the older anticonvulsants—by inhibiting the movement of ions across the neural membrane. They are useful for relieving neuropathic pain. Local anesthetics can be given:

- Topically: Local anesthetic gels and patches have been used to prevent the pain associated with needle stick and other minor procedures. Both gel and patch (Lidoderm) versions of lidocaine have been shown to reduce the pain of postherpetic neuropathy.
- Transmucosally: Lidocaine solutions can reduce pain associated with oral mucositis.
- Parenterally: Administering IV lidocaine at 1 to 5 mg/kg (maximum 500 mg) over 1 hour, followed by a continuous infusion of 1 to 2 mg/kg/h has been reported to reduce intractable neuropathic pain in patients in inpatient palliative care and home hospice settings.
- Spinally: Epidural or intrathecal lidocaine or bupivacaine delivered with or without an opioid can reduce neuropathic pain.

N-Methyl-D-Aspartate Antagonists

Antagonists to NMDA are believed to block the binding of excitatory amino acids, such as glutamate, in the spinal cord. Ketamine, a dissociative anesthetic, is believed to relieve severe neuropathic pain by blocking NMDA receptors. A recent systematic review concluded that although limitations in the data exist, ketamine may be an option for refractory cancer pain.[11] Routine use often is limited by cognitive changes, hallucinations, and other adverse effects, although small studies suggest that gradual upward titration may prevent these effects. Topical ketamine, usually in combination with amitriptyline and baclofen, may be useful for neuropathic conditions due to cancer treatment.

Bisphosphonates

Bisphosphonates inhibit osteoclast-mediated bone resorption and alleviate pain related to metastatic bone disease and multiple myeloma.[12]

- Pamidronate disodium reduces pain, hypercalcemia, and skeletal morbidity associated with breast cancer and multiple myeloma. Dosing is generally repeated every 4 weeks, and the analgesic effects occur in 2 to 4 weeks.

- Zoledronic acid and ibandronate have been shown to relieve pain due to metastatic bone disease.
- Denosumab, a newer bisphosphonate, has been shown to reduce skeletal-related events associated with solid tumors, which would reduce pain associated with fractures.
- Clodronate and sodium etidronate appear to provide little or no analgesia.

Calcitonin

Subcutaneous calcitonin may be effective in the relief of neuropathic or bone pain, although studies are inconclusive. The nasal form of this drug may be more acceptable in end-of-life care when other therapies are ineffective. Usual doses are 100 to 200 IU/day subcutaneously or nasally.

Radiation Therapy and Radiopharmaceuticals

Radiotherapy can be enormously beneficial in relieving pain due to bone metastases or other lesions. In many cases, single-fraction external beam therapy can be used to facilitate treatment in debilitated patients. Targeted therapies, also referred to as radiosurgery, can be effective in selected situations. Radiolabeled agents, also described as radiopharmaceuticals, such as strontium-89 and samarium-153 have been shown to be effective at reducing metastatic bone pain.[13] Thrombocytopenia and leukopenia are relative contraindications, because strontium-89 can cause thrombocytopenia in as many as 33% of those treated and leukopenia in up to 10%. Because of the delayed onset and timing of peak effect, only those patients with a projected life span of greater than 3 months should be considered for treatment. Patients should be advised that a transitory pain flare could occur after either external beam therapy or radiolabeled agents; additional analgesics should be provided in anticipation. Goals of treatment should be clearly articulated so that patients and family members understand the role of these therapies.

Chemotherapy

Palliative chemotherapy is the use of antitumor therapy to relieve symptoms associated with malignancy. Patient goals, performance status, sensitivity of the tumor, and potential toxicities must be considered. Uses of chemotherapy to improve symptoms include hormonal therapy in breast cancer to relieve chest wall pain due to tumor ulceration, or chemotherapy in lung cancer to relieve dyspnea. However, in a study of patients with stage IV cancers, 69% of those with lung and 81% of those with colorectal cancers did not understand the chemotherapy was not curative. Clear discussions regarding the goals of therapy are warranted.

Other Adjunct Analgesics
Capsaicin

Topical capsaicin is believed to relieve pain by inhibiting the release of substance P. This compound has been shown to be useful in relieving pain associated with postmastectomy syndrome, postherpetic neuralgia, and postsurgical neuropathic pain in cancer. A burning sensation experienced by patients is a common reason for discontinuing therapy. A Cochrane review of low-dose topical capsaicin found this therapy unlikely to have meaningful effect. A high concentration (8%) topical capsaicin patch has been found to be effective in treating HIV-associated and other painful neuropathies.

Cannabinoids
The characterization of the cannabinoid receptors (CB1 and CB2) have increased our understanding of the role of these receptors in pain and have allowed the development of more selective agents that might provide analgesia without the central nervous system depressant effects seen with tetrahydrocannabinol (THC) alone. Evidence exists for the efficacy of some of these new selective compounds in animal models of noncancer and cancer pain.[14] Nabiximols, an oral cannabinoid spray shown to be effective in advanced cancer pain poorly responsive to opioids, has been approved in Canada and countries in Europe for the relief of neuropathic pain. However, review of existing literature evaluating the role of cannabinoids currently approved for human use suggests that these agents are moderately effective with comparable adverse effects. Questions regarding the long-term safety and regulatory implications remain. Of importance to prescribers is that although a state may have legalized marijuana, it remains a federal offense.

Baclofen
Doses usually begin at 10 mg/day, increasing every few days, for the relief of spasm-associated pain. A generalized feeling of weakness and confusion or hallucinations often occurs with doses above 60 mg/day. A small retrospective chart review of patients with neuropathic cancer pain suggested benefit from oral baclofen. Intrathecal baclofen has been used to treat spasticity and resulting pain, primarily due to multiple sclerosis and spinal cord injury, although a case report describes relief from pain due to spinal cord injury and amyotrophic lateral sclerosis.

Dexmedetomidine
An alpha-2 adrenergic agonist used primarily within intensive care or during invasive procedures, has been suggested to provide relief in intractable pain, although cost and hypotension may limit its use.

Interventional Therapies
Interventional therapies to relieve pain at end of life can be beneficial, including:

- Nerve blocks
- Vertebroplasty
- Kyphoplasty
- Radiofrequency ablation of painful metastases
- Procedures to drain painful effusions

Few of these procedures have undergone controlled clinical studies. One technique, the celiac plexus block, has been shown to be superior to morphine in patients with pain due to unresectable pancreatic cancer. Choosing one of these techniques is dependent on the availability of experts in this area who understand the special needs of palliative care patients, the patient's ability to undergo the procedure, and the patient's and family's goals of care.

Nonpharmacological Therapies

Nondrug therapies, including cognitive-behavioral techniques and physical measures, can serve as adjuncts to analgesics in the palliative care setting. The patient's and caregivers' abilities to participate must be considered when selecting one of these therapies, including their fatigue level, interest, cognition, and other factors.

Cognitive-behavioral therapy often includes:

- Relaxation
- Guided imagery
- Mindfulness meditation
- Music
- Prayer
- Reframing

Physical measures include:

- Massage
- Reflexology
- Heat/cold
- Chiropractic

Difficult Pain Syndromes

The above therapies provide relief for the majority of patients using established guidelines (see Box 2.5). Unfortunately, complex pain syndromes may require additional measures. These syndromes include breakthrough pain, pain crises, and pain control in the patient with a past or current history of substance abuse.

Breakthrough Pain

Intermittent episodes of moderate to severe pain that occur in spite of control of baseline continuous pain are common in patients with advanced disease. Breakthrough pains are common in palliative care patients, occurring a 4–5 times a day, usually without warning, and lasting moments to many minutes. The risk of increasing the around-the-clock or continuous-release analgesic dose to cover breakthrough pains is that of increasing undesirable side effects, especially sedation, once the more short-lived, episodic breakthrough pain has remitted. Guidelines for categorizing, assessing, and managing breakthrough pain are described below.

Incident Pain

Incident pain is predictably elicited by specific activities. Use a rapid-onset, short-duration analgesic formulation in anticipation of pain-eliciting

Box 2.5 Guidelines for Pain Management in Palliative Care

- Sustained-release formulations and around-the-clock dosing should be used for continuous pain syndromes.
- Immediate-release formulations should be made available for breakthrough pain. Each breakthrough dose is usually 10%–20% of the 24-h dose of the sustained-release formulation. Thus, as the sustained-release dose increases, so does the immediate-release dose.
- Cost, convenience, and availability of medications (and other identified issues influencing compliance) are highly practical and important matters that should be taken into account with every prescription.
- Anticipate, prevent, and treat predictable side effects and adverse drug effects.
- Titrate analgesics based on patient goals, requirements for supplemental analgesics, pain intensity, severity of undesirable or adverse drug effects, measures of functionality, sleep, emotional state, and patients'/caregivers' reports of impact of pain on quality of life.
- Monitor patient status frequently during dose titration.
- Discourage use of mixed agonist–antagonist opioids.
- Be aware of potential drug–drug and drug–disease interactions.
- Recommend expert pain management consultation if pain is not adequately relieved within a reasonable amount of time after applying standard analgesic guidelines and interventions.
- Know the qualifications, experience, skills, and availability of pain management experts (consultants) within the patient's community before they may be needed.

These basic guidelines and considerations will optimize the pharmacological management of all patients with pain, particularly those in the palliative care setting.

activities or events. Educate patients and family members regarding the need to administer short-acting opioids approximately 30–60 minutes prior to the activity to prevent pain.

Spontaneous Pain
Spontaneous pain is unpredictable and not temporally associated with any activity or event. These pains are more challenging to control. The use of adjuvants for neuropathic pains may help to diminish the frequency and severity of these types of pain (Table 2.4). Otherwise, immediate treatment with a potent, rapid-onset opioid analgesic is indicated.

End-of-Dose Failure
End-of-dose failure describes pain that occurs toward the end of the usual dosing interval of a regularly scheduled analgesic. This results from declining blood levels of the around-the-clock analgesic before administration or uptake of the next scheduled dose. Appropriate questioning and use of pain diaries will assure rapid diagnosis of end-of-dose failure.

Bone Pain

Pain due to bone metastases or pathological fractures can include extremely painful breakthrough pain, often associated with movement, along with periods of somnolence when the patient is at rest. As a result, malignant bone pain is highly correlated with functional impairment. Current treatment of bone pain includes:

- Corticosteroids
- Bisphosphonates
- Radiotherapy or radionuclides
- Long-acting opioids along with short-acting opioids
- Vertebroplasty or kyphoplasty—may stabilize the vertebrae if tumor invasion leads to instability

Pain Crisis

When confronted by a pain crisis, the following considerations will be helpful:

- Differentiate terminal agitation or anxiety from "physically" based pain, if possible. Terminal symptoms unresponsive to rapid upward titration of an opioid may respond to benzodiazepines (e.g., lorazepam, midazolam).
- Make sure that drugs are getting absorbed. The only route guaranteed to be absorbed is the IV route. Although invasive routes of drug delivery are to be avoided unless necessary, if there is any question about oral or transdermal absorption of analgesics or other necessary palliative drugs, parenteral access should be established.
- Preterminal pain crises that respond poorly to basic approaches to analgesic therapy merit consultation with a pain management consultant as quickly as possible. Radiotherapeutic, anesthetic, or neuroablative procedures may be indicated.

Management of Refractory Symptoms at the End of Life

Sedation at the end of life is an important option for patients at home or in hospital with intractable pain, delirium, dyspnea, or other symptoms. The most commonly employed agents include benzodiazepines, including midazolam or lorazepam, barbiturates, and in some cases, propofol. Palliative sedation is best delivered under the guidance of experts in palliative care and is usually reserved for those patients who are expected to die within hours to days. Light sedation may first be attempted to allow communication with loved ones, although in some circumstances this may be insufficient to relieve the intractable symptoms. See volume 7 for an in-depth discussion of palliative sedation.

Ketamine

Ketamine is a potent analgesic at low doses and a dissociative anesthetic at higher doses, making it useful for some patients with refractory pain at the end of life.[11] Ketamine can be used:

- In the management of severe neuropathic pain
- As an opioid-sparing agent

Adverse effects are often dose-related and include psychotomimetic effects (hallucinations, dysphoria, and nightmares) as well as excess salivation. Haloperidol can be used to treat the hallucinations, and scopolamine may be needed to reduce the excess salivation seen with this drug.

Ketamine is commercially available in the United States only in a parenteral formulation. If the oral route is indicated, a palatable solution can be compounded or the parenteral solution ingested, usually mixed with juice or other liquids to mask the bitter taste. Because the opioid sparing effect is so pronounced, the opioid dose should be reduced by 25% to 50% when initiating ketamine (Box 2.6). More research is needed regarding the efficacy of, and adverse effects associated with, the use of ketamine for intractable pain in the palliative care population.

Box 2.6 Protocol for Using Ketamine to Treat Intractable Pain

1. The typical starting dose is 10–15 mg PO every 6 hours. Reversal of morphine tolerance may occur at low doses such as this, while management of neuropathic pain is likely to require higher doses.
   a. There is no commercially available oral product. The injectable product may be diluted from its standard concentration of 50 mg/mL or 100 mg/mL with cherry syrup or cola to mask the bitter taste when given orally.
   b. Consider decreasing long-acting opioid by 25%–50%.
2. Dosing may be increased *daily* by 10 mg every 6 hours until pain is relieved or side effects occur. Do not increase doses more frequently than every 24 hours.
   a. Major side effects include dizziness, a dreamlike feeling, and auditory or visual hallucinations. If intolerable side effects occur, ketamine should be decreased to the previous dose or discontinued. Resolution may not occur for 24 hours.
   b. Oral doses as high as 1000 mg per day have been reported in the neuropathic pain literature with average oral doses of 200 mg per day in divided doses required for pain relief.
3. Ketamine may be given intravenously or subcutaneously if the oral route is not available. A trial of 5–10 mg IV can also be considered, which may be repeated in 15–30 minutes.
   a. The starting infusion dose is 0.2 mg/kg/h, can increase by 0.1mg/kg/h every 6 hours, with upward titrations to 0.5 mg/kg/h or 800 mg in 24 hours.
   b. Consider decreasing long-acting opioid by 25%–50%
   c. The injectable solution is irritating and may require the subcutaneous needle to be changed daily.

From the Thomas Palliative Care Program, Virginia Commonwealth University, Richmond, VA; with permission.

Pain Control in People With Substance Abuse Disorders

The numbers of patients entering palliative care with a current or past history of substance abuse disorders are unknown, yet thought to be significant. As approximately one-third of the US population has used illicit drugs, it logically follows that some of these individuals will require palliative care. Therefore, all clinicians must be aware of the principles and practical considerations necessary to adequately care for these individuals.[15]

The underlying mechanisms of addiction are complex, including:

- The pharmacological properties of the drug
- Personality
- Psychiatric disorders
- Past use history
- Environmental issues
- Underlying genetic factors

Thorough assessment of the pain and their addictive disease is critical. Screening tools, such as the CAGE questionnaire (i.e., Cut down, Annoying, Guilty, Eye opener), have been found to predict long-term opioid treatment in cancer patients undergoing chemoradiation for head and neck cancer. Patients should be informed that the information will be used to help prevent withdrawal from these drugs, as well as ensure adequate doses of medications used to relieve pain.

Risk stratification can be helpful in clinical practice. Patients with substance use disorder can be categorized in the following manner:

- Individuals who used drugs or alcohol in the past but are not using them now
- Patients in a substitution program (methadone, buprenorphine) who are not using recreational drugs or alcohol
- Persons in a substitution program but who continue to actively use drugs or alcohol
- People using drugs or alcohol occasionally, usually socially
- Patients who are actively abusing alcohol or drug

A frequent fear expressed by professionals is that they will be "duped," or lied to, about the presence of pain. One of the limitations of pain management is that pain, and all its components, cannot be proven. Therefore, expressions of pain must be believed. As with all aspects of palliative care, an interdisciplinary team approach is indicated. This may include inviting addiction counselors to interdisciplinary team meetings.

- Realistic goals must be established. For example, recovery from addiction is impossible if the patient does not seek this rehabilitation. The goal in that case may be to provide a structured and safe environment for patients and their support persons.
- Comorbid psychiatric disorders are common, particularly depression, personality disorders, and anxiety disorders. Treatment of these underlying problems may reduce relapse or aberrant behaviors and may make pain control more effective.
- Nonopioids may be used, including antidepressants, anticonvulsants, and other adjuncts.

- Psychoactive drugs with no analgesic effect should be avoided in the treatment of pain.
- Tolerance must be considered; thus, opioid doses may require more rapid titration and may be higher than for patients without previous exposure to opioids.
- Requests for increasing doses may be due to psychological suffering, so this possibility must also be explored.
- Consistency in the treatment plan is essential. Inconsistency can increase manipulation and lead to staff frustration.
- Setting limits is a critical component of the care plan, and medication contracts may be indicated.
- In fact, one primary clinician may be designated to handle the pharmacological management of pain. Prescriptions may be written for 1-week intervals if patients cannot manage an entire month's supply. Prescriptions may be delivered to one pharmacy to reduce the potential for altered prescriptions or prescriptions from multiple prescribers.
- Use long-acting opioids whenever possible, limiting the reliance on short-acting drugs.
- Some have suggested requiring patients to bring in pill bottles to all clinic visits to conduct pill counts.
- Urine toxicology studies may be useful.
- Checking state prescription drug monitoring program websites for information regarding medication refills can help determine whether the patient is receiving prescriptions from multiple prescribers.
- Avoid bolus parenteral administration, although at the end of life, infusions can be effective and diversion limited by keeping no spare cassettes or bags in the home.
- Nondrug alternatives may also be suggested.

An additional complicating factor is that many people with addictive disease have limited psychological, social, and financial resources. Part of the reason for self-medication may be mental illness. The lack of resources makes provision of care difficult, as many of these patients may have lost their jobs and homes and have alienated friends and family members. Innovative programs offering palliative care of homeless patients living in shelters include attention to treatment of substance abuse. Other novel programs are being proposed to allow community access to palliative care patients while limiting the potential for diversion.

Patients in recovery may be extremely reluctant to consider opioid therapy. Patients may need reassurance that opioids can be taken for medical indications, such as cancer or other illnesses. If patients currently are treated in a methadone maintenance program, continue the methadone but add another opioid to provide pain relief. Communicate with the program to ensure the correct methadone dose.

An emerging area of interest is whether opioid therapy is beneficial in chronic pain. Several well-designed studies suggest increased rates of depression, misuse, and overdose in those with chronic nonmalignant pain.[16] Long-term opioid use may lead to endocrine changes in both men and women as well as increased incidence of fractures. Additionally, the increase in prescribing of opioids for chronic pain may be contributing to the rising death rate associated with opioid misuse. Although limited data are available for those with life-threatening illnesses, as palliative care moves upstream into outpatient practices with increasing numbers of patients with chronic pain, these issues will become prominent and will require thoughtful solutions.[17]

References

1. Institute of Medicine. Relieving Pain in America: A Blueprint for Transforming Prevention, Care, Education, and Research. Washington, DC: The National Academies Press; 2011.

2. Sykes N, Thorns A. The use of opioids and sedatives at the end of life. Lancet Oncol. 2003;4(5):312–318.

3. Azoulay D, Jacobs JM, Cialic R, Mor EE, Stessman J. Opioids, survival, and advanced cancer in the hospice setting. J Am Med Dir Assoc. 2011;12(2):129–134.

4. Paice JA, Ferrell B. The management of cancer pain. CA Cancer J Clin. 2011;61(3):157–182.

5. American Pain Society. Principles of Analgesic Use in the Treatment of Acute Pain and Cancer Pain. 6th ed. Glenview: American Pain Society; 2008.

6. Caraceni A, Hanks G, Kaasa S, et al. Use of opioid analgesics in the treatment of cancer pain: evidence-based recommendations from the EAPC. Lancet Oncol. 2012;13(2):e58–e68.

7. Paice JA, Von Roenn J, Hudgins JC, et al. Morphine bioavailability from a topical gel formulation in volunteers. J Pain Symptom Manage. 2008;35:314–320.

8. Davis MP. Fentanyl for breakthrough pain: a systematic review. Expert Rev Neurother. 2011;11(8):1197–1216.

9. Chou R, Cruciani RA, Fiellin DA, Compton P, Farrar JT, Haigney MC, et al. Methadone safety: a clinical practice guideline from the American Pain Society and College on Problems of Drug Dependence, in collaboration with the Heart Rhythm Society. J Pain. 2014;15(4):321–337.

10. Twycross R, Sykes N, Mihalyo M, Wilcock A. Stimulant laxatives and opioid-induced constipation. J Pain Symptom Manage. 2012;43(2):306–313.

11. Bredlau AL, Thakur R, Korones DN, Dworkin RH. Ketamine for pain in adults and children with cancer: a systematic review and synthesis of the literature. Pain Med. 2013;14(10)1505–1517.

12. Lopez-Olivo MA, Shah NA, Pratt G, Risser JM, Symanski E, Suarez-Almazor ME. Bisphosphonates in the treatment of patients with lung cancer and metastatic bone disease: a systematic review and meta-analysis. Support Care Cancer. 2012;20(11):2985–2998.

13. Ogawa K, Washiyama K. Bone target radiotracers for palliative therapy of bone metastases. Curr Med Chem. 2012;19(20):3290–3300.

14. Bostwick JM, Reisfield GM, DuPont RL. Clinical decisions: medicinal use of marijuana. NEJM. 2013;368(9):866–868.

15. Kircher S, Zacny J, Apfelbaum SM, et al. Understanding and treating opioid addiction in a patient with cancer pain. J Pain. 2011;12(10):1025–1031.

16. Edlund MJ, Martin BC, Devries A, Fan MY, Braden JB, Sullivan MD. Trends in use of opioids for chronic noncancer pain among individuals with mental health and substance use disorders: the TROUP study. Clin J Pain. 2010;26(1):1–8.

17. Paice J, Von Roenn J. Under- or overtreatment of cancer pain: How to achieve proper balance. J Clin Oncol. 2014; 32(16):1721–1726.

Chapter 3

Nausea and Vomiting

Kimberley Chow and Daniel Cogan

Nausea and vomiting are symptoms commonly experienced by patients with chronic and advanced disease. These highly distressing symptoms may be directly or indirectly related to disease and can have a significant impact on both the physiological and psychological well-being of patients. Physiologic repercussions of poorly controlled nausea and vomiting include:

- Metabolic disturbances
- Malnutrition
- Electrolyte imbalances
- Impairment of functional ability
- Unnecessary hospitalizations
- Emergency room visits
- Interruptions in disease-related treatment regimens

Psychologically, nausea and vomiting whether experienced together or separately, can cause:

- Distress
- Anxiety
- Fear
- Erosion of one's quality of life
- Strain on caregivers

To date, the majority of research on nausea and vomiting addresses the oncology population, focusing largely on treatment-induced nausea and vomiting in patients receiving chemotherapy for either curative or palliative purposes. For cancer patients receiving treatment, nausea, vomiting, and retching are among some of the most distressing symptoms reported. Despite advances in antiemetic therapies, nausea continues to be ranked as one of the most severe and distressing side effects of chemotherapy. As the palliative care integration model has shifted to be recommended as early as diagnosis, it is important to emphasize that proper palliation of these bothersome symptoms can help patients continue on with disease-targeted therapies with the aim of disease response or control.

Unfortunately, the literature on the assessment and management of nausea and vomiting in the noncancer population and in cancer patients experiencing these symptoms from causes other than chemotherapy or from terminal illness is lacking. Given the nature of current evidence-based literature, this chapter will use advanced cancer patients as a model for assessment and treatment of nausea and vomiting, which can then be extrapolated for use in other patients with advanced nononcologic diseases.

Epidemiology of Nausea and Vomiting in Palliative Care

A strong understanding of symptom prevalence in different diseases will allow clinicians to anticipate problems for the patient, develop a well-rounded plan of care, educate clinical staff, and plan for appropriate services.[1]

Cancer Population

Prevalence of nausea and vomiting in patients with advanced cancer has been reported at between 21% and 68% and is described by patients as one of the most dreaded side effects of cancer treatment. Research on nausea and vomiting over the past 25 years has led to steady improvements in the control of chemotherapy-induced nausea and vomiting, with the development of serotonin (5HT-3) receptor antagonists in the 1990s being one of the most significant advances in the chemotherapy of cancer patients.[2]

- Despite these advances, approximately 70%–80% of patients receiving chemotherapy continue to experience nausea, vomiting, or both, and 10%–44% experience anticipatory nausea, vomiting, or both.

- Oncology patients may experience these symptoms as a result of disease and/or treatment.

- The incidence, prevalence, and severity is related to the emetic potential of the chosen treatment regimen and specific patient variables, with some studies suggesting that the female gender and younger age are predisposing factors for chemotherapy-induced nausea and vomiting.

- Severity is also seen to increase as disease progresses and in some instances may be a predictor of shortened survival.

The data on prevalence of nausea and vomiting at end-of-life in cancer patients is mixed and may be related to cancer type and whether the patient is still receiving disease-targeted therapies. Some studies show that in certain cancer populations these symptoms become more prevalent closer to death and during the last week of life, impacting physical well-being. Meanwhile, other studies suggest that the prevalence and severity of nausea actually decreases closer to death. In some instances nausea was reported in only 17% of cancer patients at the end of life as compared with pain (45%) and anxiety (30%). Decreased prevalence may be due to underreporting and lack of standardized comprehensive assessments to facilitate symptom documentation.

Noncancer Population

Nausea and vomiting for patients with advanced illness other than cancer has received less attention, and recent research provides conflicting information. Multiple reports suggest that nausea and vomiting are experienced by people with advanced illness, but not to the degree previously reported, and not as commonly as pain, breathlessness, or fatigue, with incidence and severity worsening over time. There are also persuasive arguments that nausea is very likely to be underreported and undertreated especially for patients in long-term care settings. As in the cancer population, drawing firm conclusions regarding the epidemiology of nausea and vomiting in the noncancer advanced illness population is complicated by methodologic difficulties presented by the palliative care population and the lack of standardized symptom definition and reporting.[1]

- Studies available on noncancer patients consistently found that nausea and vomiting occur less frequently than many other measured symptoms.
- A systematic review examining daily symptom burden in end-stage chronic organ failure found the prevalence of nausea to range from 2% to 48%, which was less common than fatigue, dyspnea, insomnia, and pain.
- In multiple studies using the nine-item Edmonton Symptom Assessment Scale, nausea was the least frequently reported symptom.
- Though nausea is infrequently encountered as an acute complication of dialysis administration, 14.6% of patients with end-stage renal disease receiving dialysis experience nausea. A longitudinal study of patients with end-stage renal disease found 59% of patients experience nausea during the month before death, again suggesting an increase in incidence as one becomes more ill.

Conceptual Concerns Related to Nausea and Vomiting

To thoroughly examine the problem of nausea and vomiting in palliative care, it is important to be clear about certain concepts. Symptoms such as nausea and vomiting are composed of subjective components and dimensions unique to each patient. Symptoms are different from signs, which are objective and can be observed by the healthcare professional. Symptom occurrence is composed of the frequency, duration, and severity with which the symptom presents. Symptom distress involves the degree or amount of physical, mental, or emotional upset and suffering experienced by an individual. This is different from symptom occurrence. Lastly, symptom experience involves the individual's perception and response to the occurrence and distress of the symptom.

The terms "nausea" and "vomiting," often clinically associated, are in fact distinct concepts that are many times mistakenly used interchangeably or imprecisely, impacting the ability to assess and measure prevalence and burden.

- **Nausea** is an unpleasant feeling of the need to vomit experienced in the back of the throat and epigastrium. It is a nonobservable phenomenon that may be accompanied by autonomic symptoms such as pallor, cold sweat, salivation, and tachycardia as well as some degree of anorexia or loss of appetite. The patient often times describes the sensation as feeling "queasy" or "sick to my stomach" or may have a difficult time describing the unpleasant sensations experienced.

- **Vomiting** is a physical event that results in the forceful expulsion of gastric contents from the stomach and out of the mouth or nose through a complex reflex involving the gastrointestinal (GI) tract, diaphragm, and abdominal muscles. This may be described as "barfing," "upchucking," "heaving," "flipping," or "puking." The two should always be assessed separately.

- **Retching** is the body's attempt to vomit without the actual expulsion of material. Patients often describe this as "gagging" or "dry heaves." Nausea and vomiting should not be confused with regurgitation, rumination, or dyspepsia, syndromes that cause similar sensations in the upper abdomen but require different treatment approaches.

While there are multiple etiologies for nausea and vomiting in advanced cancer, chemotherapy-induced nausea and vomiting is one of the most common and can continue even near death as many patients remain on systemic therapy throughout the late stages of their disease.[3] Three distinct types of chemotherapy-induced nausea and vomiting have been described.

- Acute phase occurs anywhere from minutes to 1 day following chemotherapy and usually begins 4 or more hours later.
- Delayed phase usually occurs 24 hours following treatment.
- Anticipatory nausea and vomiting is a response to conditioned stimuli developed from significant nausea and vomiting during previous chemotherapy treatments and occurs even before treatment is administered.

Causes of Nausea and Vomiting

There are numerous potential causes of nausea and vomiting in cancer patients with advanced disease requiring palliative care. It is helpful to have a thorough understanding of the common causes, which can be subdivided into six clinical syndromes presented in Box 3.1.

Although the potential causes of nausea and vomiting are extensive and the frailty of the palliative care patient often precludes invasive diagnostic testing, studies have shown that it is possible to determine the underlying cause or causes for targeted therapy.[4] Approach to treatment relies heavily on identifying the symptoms present, the level of patient distress, grasping the physiologic mechanisms involved, and determining the underlying etiology, keeping in mind that causes are often multifactorial.[5] The skilled clinician will use his or her assessment to quickly identify any reasonably reversible causes that remain in line with the patient and family's goals of care.

Assessment of Nausea and Vomiting

The palliative care specialists' approach to symptom assessment and treatment requires understanding of symptom pathophysiology, which can be

Box 3.1 Common Syndromes Involving Nausea and Vomiting in the Palliative Care Population[1-5]

Biochemically/Drug-Induced

Fluid and electrolyte imbalances (e.g., hypercalcemia, hyponatremia)
Organ failure (e.g., liver, renal)
Chemotherapy
Opioids
Antibiotics
Anticonvulsants
SSRI antidepressants

Gastric Stasis

Carcinoma of stomach
Ascites
Opioid related
Anticholinergic drugs
Peptic ulcers

Gastrointestinal Obstruction/Irritation

Cancer related
Esophagitis
Peptic ulcers
Gastric distention or compression
Delayed gastric emptying
Bowel obstruction
Constipation
Biliary obstruction
Intra-abdominal secondaries (e.g., peritoneal disease)
Adhesions
Treatment related (e.g., chemotherapy, radiation)
Infection (e.g., cryptosporidiosis)
Medication (e.g., aspirin, NSAIDs)

Increased Intracranial Pressure

Cerebral edema
Intracranial tumor
Intracranial bleeding
Meningeal disease

Vestibular

Opioid induced
Cerebral secondaries
Motion sickness

(continued)

Box 3.1 (Continued)

Psychological

Fear

Anxiety

Anticipatory

NSAIDs = nonsteroidal antiinflammatory drugs; SSRIs = selective serotonin reuptake inhibitors

obtained from the patient's history, physical exam, and diagnostic test results. It is rare that patients present with nausea and vomiting as a first sign of advanced cancer. Generally, patients who complain of this symptom complex have a well-documented history of their disease, including diagnosis, prior treatment, and sites of metastases. Regardless, a focused exam when a patient is complaining of nausea and vomiting is needed to narrow down the list of differential diagnoses that may include, but are not limited to, drug-related adverse effects, uremia, infection, anxiety, constipation, gastric irritation, and proximal gastrointestinal obstruction.

- History of present illness and review of systems may include pattern of symptoms, possible triggers (e.g., medications, meals, movement, position, smells), presence of epigastric pain, dysphagia, thirst (seen with hypercalcemia), hiccups (seen with uremia), heartburn, and constipation.

- Physical examination should include an oral assessment for thrush or mucositis and assessment of abdomen, bowel sounds, and rectum for signs of obstruction, constipation, or impaction.

- Laboratory studies may help rule out organ dysfunction, infection, and electrolyte imbalances; radiographic exams should only be ordered if indicated to guide treatment decisions.

There are several measurement tools that may be used to assess one or more of the components of nausea and vomiting. Some tools provide a global measure while others measure a single component of the nausea and vomiting. Instruments may involve checklists, visual analog scales, patient interviews, or Likert scales; almost all involve self-report by the patient. The most commonly used tools with reliability and validity reproducible in research studies are shown in Table 3.1.

Treatment of Nausea and Vomiting

Management of nausea and vomiting requires a combination of both pharmacological and nonpharmacological approaches. Understanding the cause(s) of nausea and vomiting is crucial as it allows proper selection of treatment regimens. Often times the cause is multifactorial, requiring multiple interventions used concurrently. Investigations to rule out potentially

Table 3.1 Tools to Measure Nausea and Vomiting		
Instrument	**Type**	**Reliability/Validity**
Visual Analog Scale (VAS)	100-mm line, with anchor descriptors at each end	Reliability is a strength
Morrow Assessment of Nausea and Emesis (MANE) Rhodes Index of Nausea and Vomiting Form 2 (INV-2)	16 item, Likert scale (onset, severity–intensity) 8 item, Likert scale	Test/retest reliability 0.61–0.78 Split-half reliability 0.83–0.99 Cronbach's alpha 0.98 Construct validity 0.87
Functional Living Index Emesis (FLIE)	18 item, Likert scale	Content and criterion validity Internal consistency
From the National Comprehensive Cancer Network. NCCN Clinical Practice Guidelines in Oncology: Antiemesis. Version 1.2014. http://www.nccn.org/professionals/physician_gls/pdf/antiemesis.pdf. Accessed June 28, 2014.		

reversible or treatable causes such as dehydration, electrolyte imbalances, and constipation should be considered.

Pharmacological Management of Nausea and Vomiting

In the absence of an immediately reversible cause, nausea or vomiting is palliated through the combined use of pharmacological (Box 3.2) and non-pharmacological interventions.[1,3,5,6]

Prokinetic Agents: Metoclopramide, Domperidone, Cisapride, Erythromycin
Prokinetic medications alleviate nausea and vomiting by stimulating motility of the upper GI tract.[1] Four potential mechanisms for this effect have been proposed: stimulation of 5HT4 receptors in the gut wall, antagonism of 5HT-3 receptors in the chemoreceptor trigger zone (CTZ) and gut, activation of motilin receptors, and release of the "dopaminergic brake" on gastric emptying. At higher doses metoclopramide has antiemetic activity due to D2 receptor antagonism in the CTZ, and thus has a side-effect profile similar to antipsychotic medications, including extrapyramidal symptoms.

Box 3.2 Classes of Antiemetics
Prokinetic agents
Dopamine receptor antagonists
Antihistaminic agents
Selective 5HT-3 receptor antagonists
Corticosteroids
Benzodiazepines
Anticholinergic agents
Octreotide
Cannabinoids
Substance P antagonists (NK-1 receptor antagonists)

The only prokinetic agent currently available for use in the United States is metoclopramide. Metoclopramide is specifically indicated in the setting of gastric stasis, and is typically administered before meals. Higher doses are necessary to achieve central dopamine blockade in the CTZ. Reduced doses are recommended for patients with renal impairment and the elderly. Metoclopramide is contraindicated in the presence of complete bowel obstruction, GI hemorrhage, or perforation and immediately postoperatively.

The macrolide antibiotic erythromycin has also been identified as a prokinetic medication due to its motilin receptor stimulation, and it has been shown to be effective in treating diabetic gastroparesis. It is given at a dose of 250 mg orally three time daily or 250–500 mg daily intravenously. Side effects include hepatotoxicity and QTc prolongation.

Dopamine Receptor Antagonists: Butyrophenones, Phenothiazines, Atypical Antipsychotics

There are two classes of antidopaminergic medications that are effective antiemetics: butyrophenones and phenothiazines. Though these medications are also categorized as antipsychotics, the antiemetic doses of these drugs are typically lower than the antipsychotic doses. These medications achieve their antiemetic effect through dopamine blockade in the CTZ. With the exception of haloperidol, these medications have a broad spectrum of activity, antagonizing histaminic, muscarinic, serotonergic, and/or alpha-adrenergic receptors. These medications share a common side-effect and adverse-effect profile, including sedation, hypotension, anticholinergic effects, dystonias, extrapyramidal symptoms, QTc prolongation, and rarely neuroleptic malignant syndrome. The sedating effect may be considered beneficial when caring for patients close to death. Dose reduction and caution with elderly patients is recommended for all dopamine antagonists.

Butyrophenones: Haloperidol, Droperidol

Droperidol and haloperidol are drugs in the butyrophenone class, acting primarily as a dopamine antagonist. They achieve their antiemetic effect by binding to the D2 receptors in the CTZ. Haloperidol is less sedating than antipsychotics of the phenothiazine class. Because of its direct antidopaminergic activity, haloperidol should not be given to patients with Parkinson's disease. Consensus-based recommendations advocate the use of haloperidol to treat nausea and vomiting caused by chemical or metabolic causes. Citing its effectiveness in treating nausea as well as delirium and hallucinations, researchers identified haloperidol as one of four essential drugs needed for quality care of the dying in an international survey of palliative care clinicians. The FDA has issued black box warnings for both drugs because of concerns related to prolonged QTc.

Phenothiazines: Prochlorperazine, Chlorpromazine, Levomepromazine

Phenothiazines possess a broader spectrum of activity compared with haloperidol, blocking histaminic, muscarinic, serotonergic, and/or alpha-adrenergic receptors in addition to dopamine blockade. Their broad spectrum of activity is reflected in their numerous side effects including sedation, hypotension, anticholinergic effects, dystonias, extrapyramidal symptoms, QTc prolongation, leukopenia, and lowered seizure thresholds. The availability of oral, rectal suppository, parenteral, and sustained-release formulations offers flexibility of administration in the outpatient setting, an important consideration in the palliative care population. No randomized controlled trials examining the use of levomepromazine to treat nausea and vomiting in palliative care were identified in a recent review. Levomepromazine is not registered for use in the United States.

Atypical Antipsychotics
Olanzapine is an atypical antipsychotic that blocks dopaminergic, serotonergic, histaminic, and muscarinic receptors. It has been used as a second-line antiemetic for patients with refractory nausea, with efficacy shown in small uncontrolled studies. Olanzapine causes fewer extrapyramidal symptoms than other antipsychotics and does not usually cause QTc prolongation. In a small case series, olanzapine was effective in treating nausea refractory to other treatments.

Antihistaminic Agents: Promethazine, Cyclizine, Meclizine, Hydroxyzine, Diphenhydramine
The first generation of piperazine antihistamines have recognized antiemetic properties related to H1 receptor blockade in the vomiting center, CTZ, and vestibular nuclei. Due to their action in the inner ear, antihistamines are specifically indicated for nausea and vomiting associated with movement, dizziness, or vertigo.

- Diphenhydramine is often used in combination protocols to minimize the development of extrapyramidal side effects when dopamine antagonists are used. Adverse effects include sedation, dizziness, extrapyramidal symptoms, headache, anticholinergic effects, and lowered seizure threshold.
- Cyclizine is an H1-antihistaminic anticholinergic medication. It achieves its antiemetic effect by decreasing excitability in the inner ear labyrinth, blocking conduction in the vestibular-cerebellar pathways, and directly inhibiting the H1 receptor in the vomiting center. It is recommended for use when nausea or vomiting is caused by elevated intracranial pressure, motion sickness, pharyngeal stimulation, or mechanical bowel obstruction, and is less sedating than promethazine.

These medications also have some anticholinergic activity, which can be beneficial when treating bowel obstruction. Cyclizine has greater anticholinergic activity than promethazine, and is less sedating than scopolamine. This same anticholinergic activity may reverse the effect of prokinetic drugs such as metoclopramide.

Selective 5HT-3 Receptor Antagonists: Ondansetron, Granisetron, Tropisetron, Dolasetron, Palonosetron
Serotonin antagonists achieve their antiemetic effect by antagonizing 5HT-3 receptors centrally in the CTZ and vomiting center and peripherally in the gut wall.

- There is strong evidence to support their use in the prevention of chemotherapy-induced and radiation-induced nausea and vomiting, and their effect is enhanced by the addition of dexamethasone.

- There is a lack of evidence to support their use outside of this indication, and consensus guidelines recommend their use for chemical causes of nausea and vomiting, vomiting refractory to dopamine antagonists, or when nausea is thought to result from massive release of serotonin from enterochromaffin cells, such as bowel obstruction and renal failure.
- Due to their narrow mechanism of action compared with other antiemetics, the serotonin antagonists have a milder and more predictable side-effect profile, with constipation being the most common and significant side effect.

Corticosteroids

Though the mechanism of action that produces the antiemetic effect is not well understood, there is strong evidence to support the use of corticosteroids in multidrug combination prophylactic antiemetic treatment during chemotherapy and radiation therapy.

- It may be used to treat nausea stemming from increased intracranial pressure related to intracranial tumors, hypercalcemia of malignancy, or malignant pyloric stenosis.
- Dexamethasone enhances the efficacy of 5HT-3 receptor blockers, NK-1 blockers, and metoclopramide in the prevention of chemotherapy-induced nausea and vomiting.
- In nausea and vomiting caused by bowel obstruction corticosteroids may help to resolve the obstruction.

Side effects are well documented, with significant adverse effects on nearly all organ systems, especially with long-term use. Short-term adverse effects include hyperglycemia, insomnia, and psychosis.

Benzodiazepines

Benzodiazepines act on the GABA receptors of the cerebral cortex. Lorazepam may be used alone when the intent is to treat anticipatory nausea, due to its temporary amnestic effect, or when anxiety is a contributing factor to nausea or vomiting. Benzodiazepines have been shown to be effective to treat nausea in adult patients in combination with psychological techniques.

Anticholinergic Agents: Scopolamine, Atropine, Hyoscamine

Scopolamine (hyoscine) is a naturally occurring muscarinic antagonist, and achieves its antiemetic effect by blocking the muscarinic receptors in the vestibular nucleus and the vomiting center. It is indicated for treatment of nausea and vomiting associated with:

- Movement or dizziness
- Bowel obstruction if the obstruction cannot be resolved
- Motion sickness

Scopolamine can cause the full range of anticholinergic side effects:

- Sedation
- Constipation
- Urinary retention
- Blurry vision
- Xerostomia
- Delirium.

Elderly patients are particularly sensitive to these side effects. In the setting of imminent death, these anticholinergic properties can be used advantageously to treat excessive respiratory secretions. Anticholinergic medications are available in multiple formulations, including transdermal patches, ophthalmic drops that can be administered sublingually, and intravenous and subcutaneous injections, offering flexibility of administration in nonhospital settings.

Octreotide

Octreotide acetate is a long-acting somatostatin analog that may be helpful for nausea and vomiting associated with intestinal obstruction. It is not an antiemetic per se, but is used in treatment of intestinal obstruction. Specifically, it inhibits gastric, pancreatic, and intestinal secretions and reduces gastrointestinal motility, making it useful in cases where there is high-volume emesis.

Cannabinoids: Marijuana/Cannabis, Nabilone, Dronabinol

Marijuana is the best-known cannabinoid, dronabinol is the plant extract preparation available for prescription use. Nabilone is a semisynthetic agent. Cannabinoids are proposed to exert an antiemetic effect by binding to specific cannabinoid receptors in the brainstem and to the opioid mu receptor. In one systematic review, nabilone was found to be superior to placebo, domperidone, and prochlorperazine for management of chemotherapy-induced nausea and vomiting but not superior to metoclopramide or chlorpromazine. Cannabinoids were not found to add to benefits of 5HT-3 receptor antagonists. Another systematic review found oral nabilone or dronabinol were more effective treatments for chemotherapy-induced nausea and vomiting than dopamine antagonists, but were associated with significantly greater side effects.

Substance P Antagonists (NK-1 Receptor Antagonists)

The NK-1 receptor antagonists prevent the binding of substance P to NK-1 receptors. Aprepitant is an oral drug that acts as an NK-1 antagonist. It has been shown to be effective when combined with ondansetron and dexamethasone to prevent acute and delayed chemotherapy-induced nausea and vomiting.

Combination Protocols

The use of multidrug regimens for the management of chemotherapy-induced nausea and vomiting is supported by a strong base of evidence including multiple randomized controlled trials and clinical practice guidelines. Regimens are stratified based on the emetic potential of the chemotherapeutic medications used and differ based on treatment of acute or delayed emesis.[6] The reader is encouraged to refer to current guidelines from the National Comprehensive Cancer Network (NCCN),[5] the American Society of Clinical Oncology,[6] and the Multinational Association of Supportive Care in Cancer.[3] Despite the availability of effective means of controlling chemotherapy-induced nausea and vomiting, nausea as an adverse event is not reliably assessed, nauseated patients often do not receive treatment, and adherence to guidelines is often compromised by the omission of dexamethasone.

Home Hospice Approach to Selecting Antiemetics

Routes of administration become an important consideration in the treatment of nausea and vomiting in home care and hospice. Nauseated or vomiting patients cannot take oral medications. As opposed to hospital care, in the home it is often unrealistic to administer intravenous medications. Subcutaneous injections are far more practical to administer in the home setting, yet rely on patients or families to learn the skill of administration, which is similar in difficulty to that of insulin injection. Rectal medications are the mainstay of home antiemetic regimens, but are often not desired by patients and family caregivers. Oral dissolving tablets and intensols that can be absorbed sublingually are the best alternatives to rectal or parenteral administration of antiemetics.

To address these challenges, many hospices use topically applied gels of antiemetic medications, often in combination. Examples include ABR gel (Ativan, Benadryl, Reglan) and ABHR gel (Ativan, Benadryl, Haldol, Reglan). Early reports found these to be beneficial with minimal adverse effects. A more recent study shows that when using these formulations, lorazepam and metoclopramide are not absorbed at all, and diphenhydramine is absorbed only in trace amounts. In light of these findings, it appears that the benefit of antiemetic gels is attributable to placebo, with the lack of adverse effects due to the absence of absorption.

Nonpharmacological Approach to Nausea and Vomiting

Despite the wide selection of pharmacological interventions with varying mechanisms of action, nausea and vomiting continue to be among the most distressing side effects of chemotherapy. Even after treatment with antiemetics, the incidence of acute and delayed chemotherapy-induced nausea and vomiting has been reported to be greater than 50% and has the potential of interfering with the patient's willingness to undergo further disease-targeted treatment. In addition, anticipatory nausea and vomiting is difficult to control with pharmacological means. Due to the high incidence of nausea and vomiting in certain disease populations, the physiologic effects of uncontrolled symptoms, and the potential for negative effects on quality of life, understanding nonpharmacological approaches to symptom management and integrating them into usual care is appropriate.[7–8]

Self-Management Techniques

Self-management emphasizes patient autonomy in their own care and encourages patients and families to assume the responsibility of managing their condition. There are a variety of potentially useful self-management strategies that include psychological, cognitive, and behavioral modifications

> **Box 3.3 Self-Management Strategies for Management of Nausea and Vomiting**
>
> **Dietary Modifications***
>
> Eat smaller, more frequent meals
>
> Reduce food aromas and other strong food odors
>
> Avoid spicy, fatty, and highly salty foods
>
> Premedicate with antiemetics prior to meals
>
> Consume foods that minimize nausea and are "comfort foods"
>
> **Environmental Modifications**
>
> Avoid the sight and smell of food when not hungry
>
> Fresh air
>
> Prepare small, attractive meals
>
> Avoid strong or unpleasant odors
>
> Minimize sights, sounds, or smells that can initiate nausea
>
> **Psychological Strategies**
>
> Relaxation and meditation
>
> Deep breathing
>
> Distraction
>
> *Limited evidence exist, but experts recommend these dietary interventions in patients receiving chemotherapy to minimize nausea and vomiting.

of care (Box 3.3) and should take into account individual, health-status, and environmental factors when assessing for efficacy. While many of these interventions are not currently backed by strong evidence, they are associated with little harm and should be considered when treating nausea and vomiting in advanced disease.

Complementary and Alternative Medicine

There has been growing interest in the use of complementary and alternative medicine (CAM) alongside curative and palliative treatments. This type of medicine refers to a wide variety of therapies that can be categorized into biological (e.g., nutrition supplements and herbal medicines) and nonbiological or behavioral (e.g., music therapy, mind-body therapies, massage) interventions. Use has been associated with reduced therapy-related toxicity, improvement in disease-related symptoms, and improvement in quality of life.[7]

Patients should be educated to exercise caution before initiating certain complementary and alternative therapies because of the risk of drug interaction and adverse effects. The primary practitioner treating the patient's disease should be made aware of all conventional, complementary, or alternative modalities of treatment.

Biological Therapies

Complementary and alternative biological therapies include nutritional supplements such as vitamins, minerals, enzymes, and antioxidants as well as herbal medicines. There have been few studies performed on these specific therapies in association with their effects on nausea and vomiting in advanced disease.

- Ginger (zingiber officinale), which is a spice best known for its role as a flavoring agent for various foods. Ginger has actually been used in Ayurvedic and traditional Chinese medicine to treat GI symptoms such as nausea and excessive flatulence since the 16th century. Studies have suggested ginger's efficacy in treating postoperative nausea, motion sickness, and pregnancy-associated nausea and vomiting through a combination of antiinflammatory and antispasmodic activities. Newer studies have demonstrated the use of ginger in acute and delayed chemotherapy-induced nausea and vomiting in both the pediatric and adult population, although findings and efficacy remain mixed.
- Reported adverse effects include grade two heartburn, bruising/flushing, and rash.
- Potential adverse effects and herb-drug interactions must be understood before recommending ginger for symptom relief, as the herb has been associated with increased risk of bleeding, hypoglycemia, and increased blood-levels of tacrolimus.

Nonbiological Therapies

A large body of literature exists regarding acupuncture and acupressure for nausea and vomiting in the palliative care setting as well as in the postoperative and gynecologic population. Behavioral treatments that have specifically been recommended in guidelines for the treatment of anticipatory nausea and vomiting include progressive muscle relaxation, systematic desensitization, and hypnosis (Table 3.2).[7]

Acupuncture and Acupressure

Acupuncture is performed by trained specialists who insert fine, wire-thin needles into acupoints along a specific meridian on the body. Acupressure can be performed independent of a practitioner and differs from acupuncture in that it involves applying digital pressure or acustimulation bands, rather than needles, on designated points on the body. These techniques are thought to work by stimulating or easing energy flow. More specifically in regard to nausea and vomiting, both acupuncture and acupressure use the P6 acupoint, which is most commonly used to alleviate symptoms and is located on the anterior surface of the forearm, approximately three finger-widths away from the wrist crease.

Currently, these modalities are considered to be nonpharmacological strategies that have been evaluated as "likely to be effective" for the prevention, management, and treatment of chemotherapy-induced nausea and vomiting when used in conjunction with pharmacological interventions in mixed cancer types. A review of the current available literature favors its use in the different stages of chemotherapy-induced nausea and vomiting, however some studies have shown no statistical difference when comparing acupressure with sham and control groups. Mixed data on the effects of acupuncture and acupressure may also be due to the advances in antiemetics and a stronger focus on symptom management as a part of standard

Table 3.2 Nonbiological Complementary and Alternative Therapies

Technique	Description	Comments
Music Therapy	—Performed by credentialed professionals —Incorporated at any phase of illness —Addresses multiple dimensions of QOL —First introduced in hospice population in 1980s	—Likely to be effective —Associated with significant reduction in severity and duration of CINV —Perceived effects on autonomic nervous system —Less time and energy to implement for patients —No side effects
Aromatherapy	—Therapeutic use of essential oils primarily via inhalation of its vapors	—Oils such as peppermint and ginger have potential benefit of alleviating nausea and vomiting in postoperative and oncology patients —Studies limited by design, small sample size, varied doses and methods
Massage	—Soft tissue manipulation using touch and movement —Reduces stress and anxiety while promoting relaxation, which may lead to decreased heart rate, blood pressure, and respiratory rate	—Effectiveness not established —Variability in episodes of CINV and retching in breast cancer patients
Exercise	—Any planned, structured, and repetitive bodily movement —Incorporates cardiovascular, strength, and/or flexibility	—Effectiveness not established in a study looking at female breast cancer patients receiving chemotherapy
Cognitive Distraction	—Studied in adults and children —Learn to divert attention away from a threatening situation and toward relaxing sensations —Uses videos, games, puzzles, counting objects, deep breathing	—No side effects —Associated with decreased ANV and post-chemotherapy distress

QOL = quality of life; CINV = chemotherapy-induced nausea and vomiting; ANV = anticipatory nausea and vomiting.

From Lofti-Jam K, Carey M, Jefford M, et al. Non-pharmacologic strategies for managing common chemotherapy adverse effects: a systematic review. J Clin Oncol. 2008;26(34):5619–5629.

care. Despite the suggested benefits of acupuncture and acupressure, the limited competency of practitioners to perform these nonpharmacological techniques and limited availability of such practitioners has prevented increased use.

Progressive Muscle Relaxation

Progressive muscle relaxation allows individuals to respond to a stimulus that produces tension or anxiety by instead focusing on and isolating various muscle groups progressively up and down the body to induce relaxation. Patients will first work with trained practitioners and may be given audiotapes for home practice.

Systematic Desensitization

Commonly used to treat learning-based difficulties such as fears and phobias, systematic desensitization has proven particularly effective for treating anticipatory nausea and vomiting, as phobias may similarly develop through learned response or conditioning. The intervention works by teaching the patient how to counter a conditioned stimuli (e.g., entering the clinic, seeing the chemotherapy nurse) that normally elicits a maladaptive response (e.g., nausea and vomiting) with an incompatible response (e.g., muscle relaxation). Treatment has been documented as effective in over half of treated patients.

Hypnosis

While hypnosis was the first psychological technique used to treat and control anticipatory nausea and vomiting, very few controlled studies have been performed. Hypnosis is a behavioral intervention that teaches patients to focus their attention on thoughts or images unrelated to the actual source of distress, often using passive types of muscle relaxation and distraction. Similar to systematic desensitization, patients learn to invoke a physiologic state incompatible with nausea and vomiting. This technique has been effective mostly with children and adolescents, as they may be more readily hypnotized. Overall, studies using hypnosis for anticipatory nausea and vomiting support the benefits of this intervention as it has no undesirable side effects and requires little training.

Other Nonpharmacological Interventions

Malignant bowel obstruction is seen in approximately 3% of all advanced malignancies, particularly in the ovarian (5%–42%) and colorectal (10%–28%) cancer population, with nausea, vomiting, and pain often reported. Due to the potential of worsening symptom burden impacting quality of life up until death, potential palliative interventions to treat these types of obstructions have been studied. In one review, the authors recommend that patients admitted to hospital with symptomatic malignant bowel obstruction be offered at least one of the following interventions during admission:

- Surgery
- Stenting
- Decompression
- Percutaneous gastrostomy tube
- Nasogastric tube
- Octreotide

Invasive interventions should only proceed if in line with the patient's treatment goals and preferences and should be reserved for those who are well enough and likely to benefit. In cases where these nonpharmacological approaches are not warranted or desired, it is important to understand the pharmacological and nonpharmacological options available to alleviate nausea, vomiting, and pain at the end of life.

Nursing Interventions

Palliative care is by definition active total care; thus, it is essential that nurses have a proactive attitude toward assessing and promptly relieving nausea and vomiting for patients under their care.[8] The NCCN palliative care guidelines recommend:

- Aggressive symptom management
- Clarification of the intent of treatments
- Anticipation of the needs of patients and their families
- Involvement of the caregivers in the treatment process when appropriate

As discussed in this chapter, the NCCN guidelines emphasize the need for ongoing assessment of symptoms, therapeutic interventions, and measurement of outcomes. The palliative care nurse plays a crucial role in this aspect of care and is instrumental in promoting a collaborative approach among team members caring for their patients. Nurses in various treatment settings should be aware of the advances in the management of nausea and vomiting, changes to relevant treatment guidelines, and potential side effects of treatments being administered.

Just as vital is the role that the patient and caregivers play in managing nausea and vomiting from disease or disease treatment. Oncology patients have reported high information needs regarding self-management of treatment adverse effects. As active participants in their own care, they must be provided with the education and tools needed to confidently practice targeted symptom management and overall self-care. Personalized education plans with additional resources, including those found online, can further help patients understand how to implement the prescribed plan of care once at home. Education must include when and why to take certain antiemetics, as patients may be given multiple agents, and when to escalate symptom reporting to care providers.

For chemotherapy-induced nausea and vomiting, acute phases are usually assessed and managed in the inpatient or outpatient setting, however many patients are left to independently manage delayed nausea and vomiting, which can last up to five days post treatment. Individual characteristics may prevent patients from taking prescribed medications such as financial concerns, cost of medication, disbelief in treatment effectiveness, and perceived side effects to medication such as constipation or sedation. Likewise, certain patients may not report uncontrolled symptoms due to fear of being a "bad patient" or the perception that this is a normal part of cancer treatment.

Sitting down with the patient to address their overall environment, fears, and concerns is crucial to ensure that the steps to adequately control nausea and vomiting are achieved. Referring patients to other providers and resources such as palliative care specialists, case managers, or social workers should also be considered.

Conclusion

A major goal of palliative care is to improve quality of life by addressing suffering in all its dimensions. Nausea and vomiting profoundly affect all aspects of a person's well-being. Vigilant assessment, appropriate use and evaluation of pharmacological and nonpharmacological interventions, and appropriate patient and family education and support may avert the need for unnecessary interventions at the end of life and allow for quality of life throughout the disease trajectory up until death and through bereavement.

References

1. Glare P, Miller J, Nikolova T, et al. Treating nausea and vomiting in palliative care: a review. Clin Interv Aging. 2011;6:243–259.

2. Harris DG. Nausea and vomiting in advanced cancer. Br Med Bull. 2010;96:175–185.

3. Roila F, Herrstedt J, Aapro M, Gralla RJ, Einhorn LH, Ballatori E, et al. Guideline update for MASCC and ESMO in the prevention of chemotherapy- and radiotherapy-induced nausea and vomiting: results of the Perugia consensus conference. Ann Oncol. 2010;Suppl 5;v232–v243.

4. Gordon P, LeGrand SB, Walsh D. Nausea and vomiting in advanced cancer. Eur J Pharmacol. Eur J Pharmacol. 2014;722:187–191.

5. National Comprehensive Cancer Network. NCCN Clinical Practice Guidelines in Oncology: Antiemesis. Version 1.2014. http://www.nccn.org/professionals/physician_gls/pdf/antiemesis.pdf. Accessed June 28, 2014.

6. Basch E, Prestrud AA, Hesketh PJ, Kris MG, Feyer PC, Somerfield MR, et al. Antiemetics: American Society of Clinical Oncology clinical practice guideline update. J Clin Oncol. 2011;29:4189–4198.

7. Lofti-Jam K, Carey M, Jefford M, et al. Non-pharmacologic strategies for managing common chemotherapy adverse effects: a systematic review. J Clin Oncol. 2008;26(34):5619–5629.

8. Thompson N. Optimizing treatment outcomes in patients at risk for chemotherapy-induced nausea and vomiting. Clin J Oncol Nurs. 2012;16(3):309–313.

Chapter 4

Dysphagia, Xerostomia, and Hiccups

Constance Dahlin and Audrey Kurash Cohen

Dysphagia

Definition

Dysphagia is defined as difficulty swallowing food or liquid.[1] Swallowing impairments can threaten the safety and efficiency with which oral alimentation is maintained. Chronic difficulty swallowing can be both frustrating and frightening for patients. Because nutrition is compromised, generalized weakness, diminished appetite, and weight loss or malnutrition may ensue. Aspiration may also occur, causing pneumonia, fevers, malaise, shortness of breath and, rarely, death.

The psychological impact of dysphagia cannot be underestimated. Its development may be a pivotal symptom that prompts changing the goals of care to a more palliative nature. Life is not compatible with absence of fluid intake. Thus, when the patient can neither drink, nor eat, nor receive artificial nutrition and hydration, death becomes more imminent. The challenge in palliative care in managing dysphagia is how to ensure comfort, even at the expense of optimal nutrition and hydration.

Normal Swallowing

Understanding the physiology of normal and aberrant swallowing is critical to meeting the challenge of caring for the patient with dysphagia. Swallowing, an extremely complex physiological act, involves the passage of food or liquid from the oral cavity through the esophagus and into the stomach, where the process of digestion begins. Its exquisite timing and coordination of more than 30 pairs of muscles under both voluntary and involuntary nervous system control is extraordinary. The act of swallowing takes less than 20 seconds from the moment of bolus propulsion into the pharynx until the bolus reaches the stomach. For purposes of discussion, the act of swallowing is divided into three stages: the oral stage, the pharyngeal stage, and the esophageal stage. In reality, these stages occur simultaneously, with some melding and overlap of events.

Etiology of Dysphagia

Many conditions can cause dysphagia in patients receiving palliative care. In some cases, side effects of treatment such as radiation therapy or chemotherapy are the causative factors of dysphagia. In other cases, progressive disease leads to unsafe and inefficient swallowing. Understanding the physiological impact of the illness is critical in evaluation of the swallowing disorder and the method of management. Some commonly encountered etiological categories in palliative care are discussed below.

Neoplasms: Brain and Central Nervous System Tumors

Brain tumors are classified into primary and secondary types. Primary brain tumors are a diverse group of neoplasms arising from different cells of the brain, meninges, and central nervous system (CNS). In contrast, secondary tumors originate elsewhere in the body and metastasize to the brain. Although dysphagia is rarely the presenting symptom, swallowing problems can develop directly or indirectly as the tumor increases in size and compresses surrounding structures and can be present in as many as 85% of brain tumor patients in the last stages of life.

Extrinsic tumors located around the brainstem, as well as those originating in the skull base, may compress or invade the lower medulla. Hence, the swallowing center may be affected, with the specific swallowing impairment dependent on which cranial nerves are disrupted. In addition to direct tumor effects, swallowing and/or inability to maintain sufficient oral nutrition may be indirectly affected by depressed levels of consciousness, reduced awareness, fatigue, depression, seizures, and sarcopenia (changes to muscle bulk and strength), as well as the need for opioids that is associated with tumor progression, mass effect, and associated complications, especially in high-grade gliomas.

High-grade gliomas (glioblastomas), the most common form of malignant brain tumors, account for 16% of all primary brain tumors and carry a poor prognosis.[2] Median survival rates are 1 to 5 years with less than 5% of patients surviving 5 years post diagnosis. These tumors commonly result in seizures, altered consciousness, progressive cognitive deficits, and difficulty swallowing in the end-of-life phase. These symptoms can impact the patient's ability to take oral medications in the last weeks of life, including antiseizure or glucocorticoid medications.

Neoplasms: Head and Neck Cancer

It is estimated that there are 600,000 new cases of head and neck cancer around the globe each year. Oropharyngeal dysphagia is ubiquitous in patients with advanced-stage head and neck cancer. Dysphagia occurs both as a direct consequence of the disease as well as an immediate or delayed consequence of the treatment. These tumors occur in a variety of sites in the oral cavity, nasal cavity, sinuses, pharynx, larynx, and upper esophagus and can affect nerve supply, muscle coordination, and strength of movements involved in swallowing. Overall, the 5-year relative survival rate for all patients with head and neck cancers is 66%, although this rate is rising with the increasing prevalence of HPV-associated tumors, which are often quite curable.

Treatment approaches for advanced disease include surgery and chemoradiotherapy, depending on the cell type, location, tumor size, and presence of neck metastases. In extensive disease of the oral cavity or in cases of persistent or recurrent tumors, disfiguring surgical resection may be followed by reconstruction with a flap of tissue borrowed from another part of the body such as the fibula or radial forearm. Surgical resection can result in anatomic insult that interferes with the normal biomechanics of the oropharyngeal physiology, such as in the case of a glossectomy or mandibulectomy. Removal of all or a portion of the tongue will impact the ability to adequately chew, move the food around the mouth, and propel it into the pharynx.

Surgical treatment for advanced laryngeal cancer removes structures that are critical to airway protection and increase the risk for material to be misdirected into the airway and thus aspirated. Laryngectomy is seldom used as a first-line treatment for cancer of the larynx and has significant impact on patients' communication, but is used in cases of persistent or recurrent disease or may be considered an elective option for chronic, severe aspiration.

In the past two decades, "organ preservation" involving chemoradiation therapy has been the primary approach for treating cancers of the pharynx and larynx with the goal of sparing the organs involved in speech and swallowing. Unfortunately, "organ preservation" is not synonymous with "functional preservation." In spite of advances in treatment methods aimed at sparing normal tissue and targeted chemotherapy agents, patients suffer from significant treatment toxicities including pulmonary aspiration, mucositis, edema, xerostomia, and trismus (restricted jaw opening). Cranial neuropathies and fibrosis can affect airway protection, pharyngeal contraction, and bolus drive, and opening of the upper esophagus.

Radiation effects are progressive and commonly result in chronic dysphagia and aspiration. Swallowing becomes deliberate and determined with coughing, food getting caught, and the need for large volumes of liquid intake to combat dry mouth.

Nonoral nutritional support is required in greater than 60% of patients receiving multimodality treatment, and some patients are unable to resume an oral diet once their treatment is completed. A primary goal of therapy for these patients is to keep them eating. Some patients manage to compensate for their dysphagia with use of a prosthetic device fitted by a prosthodontist and changes in posture or diet consistencies suggested by the speech-language pathologist (SLP). Therapy to maximize jaw opening can be beneficial for patients with a condition known as trismus, the limited mobility of the mouth and jaw opening due to surgery or radiation that interferes with mastication. With local disease progression and distant metastasis, facial edema and pain increase and eating and drinking become chronically uncomfortable, effortful, and difficult.

Neoplasms: Malignant Esophageal Tumors

The incidence of malignant esophageal tumors in the United States was expected to rise to over 17,000 new cases in 2013. Esophageal carcinoma can arise either from squamous cells of the mucosa or as adenocarcinomas of the columnar lining of Barrett's epithelium. In the last several decades adenocarcinoma has increased and is now four to five times more prevalent in newly diagnosed cases. Tumors of the squamous cell type are generally located in the upper or midesophagus, while tumors of the adenocarcinoma type are located more distally.

Treatment options are more numerous and survival rates are much higher when the disease is detected early. Unfortunately, symptom presentation usually occurs late in the disease, resulting in diagnosis of advanced malignancy. Patients commonly report:

- Weight loss
- Progressive dysphagia with solid foods rather than liquids
- Throat pain
- Vomiting
- Intractable cough, which may indicate extension of the tumor to the mediastinum or trachea

Symptom presentation for patients with adenocarcinoma is gastroesophageal reflux disease rather than dysphagia and weight loss. Survival rates are reported to be between 10% and 20% at 5 years, and thus, palliative care is the foundation of management for this disease.

If diagnosed early, esophagectomy or esophagogastrectomy may be the treatment of choice, even with a 5% mortality rate and a 64% complication rate following these procedures. In cases of unresectable advanced disease, symptomatic relief of dysphagia and pain can be accomplished by external beam radiation therapy, brachytherapy, esophageal dilation, chemotherapy, placement of a plastic or wire mesh esophageal stent to open the lumen of the esophagus, or laser tumor ablation. Concomitant radiation therapy and chemotherapy is more effective than radiation alone for localized esophageal cancer and is increasingly being used for palliative treatment. Esophageal perforation during laser surgery or dilation and migration of the esophageal stents are potential complications from palliative procedures. Each of these treatments is associated with considerable side effects that can make swallowing painful and difficult, including esophagitis, mucositis, xerostomia, loss of taste, and lymphedema.

Neoplasms: Non–Head and Neck

Oncology patients may develop transient or persistent oropharyngeal dysphagia due to a wide range of issues including:

- Presence of tumor
- Radiation
- Cytotoxic effects of chemotherapy
- Cancer-related weakness and fatigue
- Neurologic or respiratory compromise
- Left recurrent laryngeal nerve paralysis (usually from intrathoracic tumors)
- Surgical procedures such as hilar lung tumor resection, mediastinal lymph node biopsy, and thyroidectomy
- Esophagitis as a result of radiation therapy to the mediastinum
- Mucositis of the oral, pharyngeal, and/or esophageal mucosa due to chemotherapy
- Herpes simplex virus or varicella zoster infection during periods of myelosuppression after chemotherapy
- Cancer cachexia

Progressive Neuromuscular Diseases

Motor Neuron Disease

Motor neuron diseases, of which the most common is ALS, are encountered with unfortunate regularity in patients on a palliative care service. A rapidly progressive, degenerative and terminal disease, ALS involves the motor neurons of the brain and spinal cord. One-quarter of ALS patients initially present with swallowing difficulty, while other patients begin with distal weakness that travels proximally to involve the bulbar musculature. As the disease progresses, it encompasses upper and lower motor neurons, affecting speaking, walking, writing, and ultimately the respiratory system. Respiratory failure is the usual cause of death in patients with ALS because of weakness in diaphragmatic, laryngeal, and lingual function.

Patients generally live between 3 and 5 years after diagnosis of ALS, making a coordinated and multidisciplinary team approach part of standardized treatment, essential in caring for these patients. As respiratory muscles weaken, breathing becomes impaired, inducing poor gas exchange and hypoventilation. Typically, patients with bulbar ALS experience a reduction in tongue mobility, oral and pharyngeal muscle weakness, and fatigue with eating. They develop increasing difficulty with the ability to chew and to control material in the mouth. Nasal regurgitation of fluids and loss of control over liquids may occur, resulting in aspiration and coughing before the swallow is triggered. With disease progression, heavier foods—even pureed ones—are difficult to manipulate, resulting in significant residue in the oral cavity. Reduced pharyngeal drive also results in residue in the pharynx. Diet modifications with calorie-dense foods and postural alterations are necessary if oral intake is to continue.

Many patients reach a point where the burden of eating outweighs the pleasure; significant weight loss and frequent choking may occur. Maintenance of nutrition is further challenged by muscle atrophy and a state of hypermetabolism. Gastrostomy tube placement, if undertaken before body mass index has significantly dropped and before vital capacity drops below 50% anticipated,[3] may stabilize weight loss, prolong survival, reduce complications, and improve quality of life in some patients.

Parkinson's Disease and Parkinsonian Syndromes

Parkinson's disease (PD) is a relatively common, slow progressive disease of the CNS, marked by an inability to execute learned motor skills automatically. Classic motor symptoms include resting tremor, bradykinesia (slowness of movement) and rigidity, gait dysfunction, and postural instability. Nonmotor features may include autonomic disturbances, sleep problems, and cognitive dysfunction. The largest etiological group is idiopathic; however, Parkinson-like symptoms may occur as a result of medications, toxins, head trauma, or degenerative conditions.

Dysphagia in Parkinson's disease may occur in the oral, pharyngeal, and/or esophageal stages.[4] It is related to changes in striated muscles under dopaminergic control and in smooth muscles under autonomic control. The oral stage is associated with rigidity of the lingual musculature rather than weakness. Small-amplitude, ineffective tongue-rolling movements are observed as patients attempt to propel the boluses into the pharynx. As a result, pharyngeal swallow responses are delayed, with aspiration occurring before and during the swallow. Expectoration of aspirated material occurs via only a weak cough because of rigidity of the laryngeal musculature. Incomplete opening of the upper esophageal sphincter and esophageal dysmotility are also commonly observed in patients with PD. Even mild swallowing impairments may negatively affect quality of life for patients with PD and their caregivers, often adding to their perceived burden and worries.

In the early stages, antiparkinsonian medications such as levodopa or dopamine agonists improve flexibility and speed during swallowing. This medical therapy does not stop progression of the disease, however, and the majority of patients with PD continue to decline. In patients with dysphagia who develop severe symptoms, pharmacotherapy has a limited benefit. Dysphagia and resultant pneumonia is one of the most prevalent causes of death in patients with Parkinson's disease.

Two other progressive neuromuscular diseases include progressive supranuclear palsy (PSP) and multiple system atrophy (MSA). Progressive supranuclear palsy is often initially misdiagnosed as Parkinson's. Early development of orthostasis, falls, and vertical gaze palsy are cardinal features of PSP and distinguish it from Parkinson's disease. Patients with PSP do not respond as well as patients with Parkinson's disease to pharmacological treatment, and thus their dysphagia may be more aggressive and more life threatening.

Multiple system atrophy is a progressive neurodegenerative disorder characterized by parkinsonism, ataxia, pyramidal signs such as spasticity, and autonomic failure such as urinary dysfunction and orthostatic hypotension. Generally, most patients with MSA do not respond to levodopa treatment or respond only short-term, and thus therapy is generally symptomatic. Dysphagia onset occurs within 5 years after diagnosis with MSA-P (the parkinsonian subtype).

Myopathies

Myopathy is a neuromuscular disorder that results in muscle weakness and can be either inherited or acquired. Some causes can be treated, such as infectious, toxic, endocrine, and alcohol related. The group of myopathies, known as muscular dystrophies, is chronic and progressive, resulting in continued muscle weakness affecting oral, pharyngeal, and esophageal muscles. Oculopharyngeal muscular dystrophy (OPMD) is an autosomal dominant muscle disorder with hallmark features of a slowly progressive ptosis and dysphagia, proximal limb and facial weakness, and abnormal gait, with onset generally occurring after age 40. The leading causes of death for patients with OPMD are recurrent aspiration pneumonia and malnutrition.

Duchene's muscular dystrophy is a childhood form that generally occurs in boys before the age of 6 and results in severe dysphagia by age 12.

The dysphagic symptoms include reduced palatal elevation, weak pharyngeal contraction, reduced hyolaryngeal excursion, and reduced esophageal motility. Patients tend to have secretions that pool in their pharynx, aspiration, reflux, and poor gastrointestinal (GI) motility. Medical and drug treatments are ineffective in managing the disease, and thus treatment focuses on alleviation of symptoms. Surgically, there is some evidence that a myotomy (cutting of the upper esophageal sphincter, or UES) and/or upper esophageal dilation may be beneficial in cases of moderate/severe dysphagia to open the channel from the pharynx to the esophagus more readily.

Multiple Sclerosis

Multiple sclerosis (MS) is characterized by multifocal plaques of demyelination within the CNS. It affects approximately 400,000 people in the United States. The scattered inflammatory white-matter lesions observed in the CNS result in varying combinations of motor, sensory, and cognitive deficits. It usually follows a remitting-relapsing course that within 10 years advances to the secondary progressive form. Symptoms that affect quality of life include fatigue, spasticity, paroxysmal symptoms, pain, ataxia, bladder and bowel dysfunction, depression, cognitive problems, and dysphagia. Dysphagia occurs in 34% of end-stage MS patients and appears to be related to nonambulatory patients with brainstem impairment. Swallowing dysfunction depends on the location of the lesions. For instance, difficulties may arise with the feeding process as a result of hand tremors and spasticity. Alternatively, sclerosed plaques can be found in the cortex and the brainstem and can affect cranial nerves, whereby people are unable to perform certain activities.

Dementia

Dementia encompasses Alzheimer's disease, cumulative brain damage from multiple small cerebral infarcts (vascular dementia), advanced Parkinson's or Huntington's disease, frontotemporal dementia, Lewy body disease, and brain damage from excessive and chronic alcohol. Symptoms include progressive memory loss, poor awareness, loss of language abilities, inactivity, agitation, and confusion. Dysphagia in patients with dementia is extremely prevalent, and may be as high as 93%. As a result, patients with dementia frequently develop pneumonia, malnutrition, and dehydration particularly in the advanced stages of the disease. Aspiration and weight loss increase mortality risk, irrespective of the dementia severity. Since early identification of dysphagia may reduce the onset and severity of these symptoms, frequent screening and monitoring of swallowing function is suggested. Swallowing and feeding problems that arise in the late stages of dementia are not reversible, although treating concomitant infections, metabolic disarray, and/or dehydration may result in improved functioning.[5]

The different types of dementia and their varying trajectories result in an unspecific dysphagia. However, common attributes include the inability to independently self-feed and inability to focus for the duration of meal times. With disease progression, patients may not engage in the task of eating and swallowing at all. They may hold food in their mouth for prolonged periods without mastication or bolus formation, especially with uniformly textured foods such as pureed items or bland foods. This often occurs when a swallowing dyspraxia (poor motor planning) of advanced dementia occurs. Decreased consciousness and sedation predispose patients to both food and liquid aspiration. Additionally, sensory impairments and lack of attention reduce the ability to control the bolus in the mouth, resulting in aspiration from premature spillage before the pharyngeal swallow has been elicited. Moreover, behaviors such as distraction or agitation may prolong the feeding time and hence reduce the amount of nutrition and hydration received. As dementia progresses, patients develop a lack of desire to eat and reduced appetite as a hallmark feature of late-stage dementia.

There is growing consensus among medical care providers that in advanced and late-stage dementia a palliative care approach, particularly foregoing the use of feeding tubes, is appropriate. In 2013, two new position statements were published addressing the growing evidence of the burdens associated with tube feeding in patients with advanced dementia. The revised 2013 statement by American Geriatrics Society (AGS) states, "Percutaneous feeding tubes are not recommended for older adults with advanced dementia. Careful hand feeding should be offered; for persons with advanced dementia, hand feeding is at least as good as tube feeding for the outcomes of death, aspiration pneumonia, functional status and patient comfort. Tube feeding is associated with agitation, increased use of physical and chemical restraints, and worsening pressure ulcers."[5] A special task force from the American Academy of Hospice and Palliative Medicine (AAHPM) recommended against placing feeding tubes in patients with advanced dementia. Rather, focus should be on assisted feeding for comfort and human interaction.

Medical Etiologies
Systemic Dysphagia

The broadest category of causes of dysphagia includes inflammatory and infectious factors, which affect oral, pharyngeal, and esophageal stages of swallowing. Autoimmune inflammatory disorders can affect swallowing in either specific organs or the immune system as a whole. This category of diseases includes polymyositis, scleroderma, inflammatory myopathy, and secondary autoimmune diseases. Sometimes, intrinsic obstruction is observed, such as in Wegener's granulomatosis. With other disorders, there is external compression, as in sarcoidosis; abnormal esophageal motility, as in scleroderma; or inadequate lubrication, as in Sjögren's syndrome.

Poor esophageal motility restricts patients to small meals of pureed or liquid substances, resulting in long-drawn-out eating. Weight loss is frequent, and gastroesophageal reflux can result from poor esophageal peristalsis Immunocompromised hosts, such as patients with AIDS, patients who have undergone chemotherapy, and patients on steroid therapy, are prone to candida esophagitis. Dysphagia for solids is greater than for liquids, and patients frequently complain of food getting caught. Heartburn, nausea, and vomiting are other common complaints.

General Deconditioning, Aging, and Chronic Illness

Multisystem progressive diseases, including end-stage chronic obstructive pulmonary disease (COPD), coronary artery disease, congestive heart failure (CHF), and chronic renal failure, cause insidious weakness. Weight loss in these patients is a common consequence because of reduced endurance for activities of daily living, including eating and swallowing. Body wasting, or cardiac cachexia, is a serious complication of CHF and associated with poor prognosis.

Frail elders, or elderly with "failure to thrive," constitute another set of patients who may present with chronic dysphagia. Aging can result in changes to the muscle bulk and strength (sarcopenia) and tissue elasticity in the tongue and pharynx, resulting in reduced ability to push the bolus through.[6] Additionally, aging affects the larynx; specifically the vocal folds may not close sufficiently or quickly enough to protect the airway. Sensorimotor changes may occur that impact salivary production, taste, and smell.

Dysphagia may present in hospitalized medical patients who may already have cachexia, loss of muscle mass, significantly compromised pulmonary systems that impede airway protection, and/or general weakness and deconditioning from a multitude of illnesses and lengthy hospital stays.[7] In a fragile and immunocompromised condition, there is a higher risk for suffering from pulmonary infections, poor outcomes from aspiration, and fatigue, which impacts the ability to sustain appropriate nutrition. Moreover, this group of hospitalized medical patients is prone to negative outcomes from dysphagia, including increased length of hospital days and increased risk of mortality. Particularly, difficulty in completing oral care due to a low level of consciousness and/or the presence of an endotracheal tube can promote colonization of oral bacteria in the hospitalized patient. If aspiration of colonized oropharyngeal contents occurs (secretions, vomitus, food/liquid mixed with colonized secretions) it can be a major contributor to aspiration pneumonia.

Dysphagia as a Side Effect of Medications

There are 160 known medications with dysphagia specified as a potential adverse effect. Any medication should be reviewed to determine whether it contributes to or causes a dysphagia. Medications may affect all stages of swallowing including lubrication of the oral cavity and pharynx, taste and smell, reduced coordination or motor function, impaired consciousness, GI dysfunction, and local mucosal toxicity.

- Antipsychotic or neuroleptic medications can produce extrapyramidal motor disturbances, resulting in impaired function of the striated musculature of the oral cavity, pharynx, and esophagus. Long-term use of antipsychotics may result in tardive dyskinesia, with choreiform tongue movements affecting the coordination of swallowing. Delayed swallow initiation is a reported side effect of some neuroleptic medications. Use of antipsychotic medications within the hospital setting has been found to result in impaired swallowing function with worsening of swallowing function as dosage increases.

- Anticonvulsants such as phenobarbital, carbamazepine, and phenytoin may all have adverse effects and may impact CNS functioning, drowsiness, and motor incoordination.
- Antihistamines and antidepressants may reduce taste and smell and decrease lubrication. Many of these medications can also alter GI motility, cause mucositis, or increase reflux including antipsychotics, antidepressants, and antihistamines.

Role of the Speech-Language Pathologist in End-of-Life Care

Speech-language pathologists are the expert specialists in assessment and management of communication and oropharyngeal swallowing disorders. They play a critical role as part of the multidisciplinary team for palliative care patients and can help to add comfort and maximize quality of life, as well as educate the patient and family and help prepare them to deal with the progressive symptoms of dysphagia that may accompany the disease. The SLP can use his/her knowledge to carefully explain the swallowing process and any impairments, evaluate empirical data to determine swallowing potential, prognosticate to assist in decision-making, and guide families and caregivers in safe feeding methods. The SLP provides further assistance to the care team by implementing the most effective strategies to best communicate with a patient who has impaired communication ability, including speaking valves for the patient with a tracheostomy and/or assistive and augmentative communication devices. Such interventions can improve the patient's ability to participate in decision-making and in expressing their wishes, and in maintaining social connections—hallmark features of palliative care.

A comprehensive swallow evaluation done by the SLP includes:

- A thorough review of the patient's medical history and presenting complaint
- Evaluation of alertness, hemodynamic stability, and oromotor functioning
- Observation of swallowing of various liquid and solid food consistencies, depending on the safety and appropriateness
- An instrumental swallow evaluation (via video fluoroscopy or endoscopy), if indicated

Because of their expertise in swallowing, SLPs can assist patients and families during the decision-making process of alternative hydration and nutrition with a focus on comfort, maintaining quality of life, and upholding the patient's wishes.

Speech-language pathologists who care for palliative care patients must carefully weigh what will benefit the patient and what will be burdensome. They must understand the underlying disease processes while attending to the individual, spiritual, and emotional issues, and must be skilled in biomedical ethics and legal issues and highly sensitive to the psychosocial ramifications of altering oral diets.

Assessment of Dysphagia

Evaluation of dysphagia in patients receiving palliative care is best accomplished within a multidisciplinary framework. Approaching the evaluation of swallowing in the terminally ill patient demands a holistic view and reaches beyond the physiology of deglutition. While aspiration of food or liquid could realistically evolve into pneumonia, paradoxically, committing a patient to nonoral feeding or non per os (NPO) is also fraught with complications. It therefore behooves caregivers to carefully consider the multiple parameters in decision-making about oral nutrition in the terminally ill patient.

For the patient with a serious and life-limiting illness, the goals of the swallowing evaluation are to: (1) identify the underlying physiological nature of the disorder, (2) determine whether any short-range interventions can alleviate the dysphagia, and (3) collaborate with the patient, family, and caregivers on the safest and most efficacious method of nutrition and hydration.

Balancing the safety and health of the patient with quality of life issues is integral to the assessment. Eliciting a description of the patient's complaints about swallowing, current eating habits, appetite, and diet is critical to understanding the physiological basis of the problem and to integrating these hypotheses with attitudes and wishes about eating and not eating. Details of disease progression and prognosis, along with the accompanying emotional and psychological impact on the patient and the family and consideration of a patient's cognitive status, alertness, and ability to follow directions are also be considered when determining the aggressiveness of a swallowing workup and treatment. The patient with a poor appetite, fatigue, and a sense of hopelessness will understandably be less compliant and less motivated to engage in a complex treatment program. Alternatively, the patient who derives much satisfaction from eating and drinking and wishes to continue with a regular diet, will not be satisfied with significant alterations in texture and consistency.

Examination of Swallowing by Direct Observation
Direct observation of the patient eating, drinking, or taking medications by a perceptive clinician can yield valuable information about the underlying disorder. As discussed previously, the SLP is vigilant for indications of chewing inefficiencies, aspiration, difficulties managing secretions, or obstruction.

Typically, the clinician assesses the patient's oral-motor and sensory function and cognitive communicative abilities, while observing the partaking of a variety of liquid and solid foods (e.g., semisolid, soft solid, and, where appropriate, food requiring mastication). Speech and voice are analyzed to assist in understanding the underlying physiology of the swallowing disorder. Functional airway protection is a critical predictor of safe swallowing and, thus, an important element of the swallowing evaluation, although it cannot be definitively discerned from clinical observation alone. Patients who have weak voices and weak respiratory force for coughing and pulmonary clearance are at risk for pulmonary compromise.

Since aspiration may be silent in up to 40% of patients with dysphagia, (e.g., present with no overt sign or symptom that material has entered into the airway such as a cough or throat clear), close attention is paid to occult signs of aspiration, including wet vocal quality or gurgliness, frequent throat clearing, delayed coughing, and oral/pharyngeal residue. Silent aspiration can only be confirmed definitively with an instrumental examination. Depending on the stage of progression of the patient's illness and overall management goals, it may be prudent to identify silent aspiration with the aim of limiting progression with behavioral strategies.

Screening of Swallowing Function

In the last several years there has been increased awareness of the need to screen swallowing and assess risk for aspiration before giving patients anything to eat or drink, including oral medications. This has been largely driven by the extensive research done on acute stroke patients and their high risk of aspiration (40%–60%), the close relationship between aspiration and aspiration pneumonia, and the evidence that shows that mortality rates in acute stroke patients with pneumonia are three times higher than in those without. As a result, since 2005, several national regulatory and safety guidelines including the Joint Commission and the American Heart Association state that all acute stroke patients should have their swallowing screened before any oral intake. Although this currently relates to acute stroke patients, there is increasing awareness of the risk of aspiration and the need to determine swallowing safety in many hospitalized patient populations.

The swallow screening is typically done by the nurse and identifies potential aspiration risk, assists in determining whether it is safe for a patient to start eating and drinking, and helps to determine whether a patient requires a full evaluation by the SLP. It cannot, however, determine an etiology or underlying physiology of the swallowing disorder and therefore cannot determine appropriate compensatory strategies, treatment, or prognosis. Additionally, the registered dietician may identify warning signs of dysphagia during a nutrition intake and request SLP involvement. If a patient is suspected of having a swallowing disorder (see Box 4.1), a comprehensive swallow evaluation should be completed.

A word of caution is needed regarding the gag reflex and oropharyngeal swallowing. The gag reflex and the pattern of neuromuscular events making up the swallow are very different, both in their innervation and in their execution. The gag reflex is a protective reflex that prevents noxious substances arising from the oral cavity or digestive tract from entering the airway. It is not elicited during the normal swallow, and its assessment is not clinically relevant to swallowing ability. In fact, 20% to 40% of normal, healthy adults do *not* have a gag reflex. In addition, the gag reflex can be extinguished or reduced by a nasogastric feeding tube, endotracheal intubation, or repeated stimulation.

Instrumental Evaluation

An instrumental swallow evaluation may be indicated to further delineate swallowing physiology, locate a specific etiology that may provide valuable information for management, assess for integrity of the swallowing anatomy and mucosa, determine effectiveness of swallowing strategies, and clarify or confirm aspiration risk. Instrumental or objective evaluations may take many forms, depending on the patient complaints and likely cause.

Box 4.1 Indications of a Swallowing Disorder

Reduced Alertness or Cognitive Impairment

Coma, heavy sedation, dementia, delirium

Inattention during eating

Impulsivity with regard to eating

Playing with food

Alterations in Attitudes Toward Eating

Refusal to eat in the presence of others

Avoidance of particular foods or fluids

Protracted meal times, incomplete meals, large amounts of fluids to flush solids

Changes in posture or head movements during eating

Laborious chewing, multiple swallows per small bites

Weight loss

Signs of Oral-Pharyngeal Dysfunction

Dysarthria or slurred, imprecise speech

Dry mouth with thick secretions coating the tongue and palate

Wet voice with "gurgly" quality

Drooling or leaking from the lips

Residual food in the oral cavity after eating

Frequent throat clearing, coughing, or choking during or immediately after meals

Nasal regurgitation

Recurrent aspiration pneumonias

Signs of Esophageal Dysfunction

Regurgitation or emesis after swallowing

Sour taste in mouth after eating

Solids caught in the chest region

Burping during/after eating

Pain on swallowing

Specific Patient Complaints

Sensation of food caught in the throat

Coughing and choking while eating

Regurgitation of solids through the nose after eating or drinking

Pain on swallowing

Food or fluid noted in tracheotomy tube

Inability to manage secretions

Drooling

Shortness of breath while chewing or after meals

Difficulty initiating the swallow

Unexplained weight loss

Protracted meal times or inability to complete a meal

Videofluoroscopic Evaluation of Swallowing

Radiographic swallowing studies are used to determine the pathology of impaired swallowing. The videofluoroscopic swallowing study (VFSS; commonly known as modified barium swallow study or MBS) examines oropharyngeal swallowing with the patient positioned upright while swallowing a variety of consistencies of barium-coated foods (liquids, semisolids, and solids) in controlled volumes. The study, completed by an SLP and radiology staff, is recorded digitally and the results are reviewed following the study for closer inspection of the anatomy and physiology. The goal of this study is not only to determine the presence or absence of aspiration but also to evaluate the effectiveness of compensatory swallowing strategies that may decrease the risk of aspiration and increase swallowing efficiency. The test is noninvasive, takes little time to administer, and provides valuable information to manage the dysphagia.

Fiberoptic Endoscopic Evaluation of Swallowing

Using fiberoptic endoscopic evaluation of swallowing (FEES), endoscopic examination of oropharyngeal swallowing can be performed at the bedside by a trained SLP. The oropharynx and larynx can be visualized transnasally while the patient is swallowing food substances dyed with food coloring. The presence of laryngeal penetration, aspiration, and pharyngeal retention can be observed; laryngeal and oropharyngeal anatomy viewed; and sensory integrity of the pharynx and larynx assessed. As with the VFSS, compensatory swallowing strategies such as postural modifications or swallowing maneuvers can be evaluated for their efficacy in the FEES. The use of the endoscope can also provide visual feedback to the patient during treatment.

Barium Swallow and Upper Gastrointestinal Study

In contrast to the VFSS, which focuses on the oropharyngeal mechanism, a barium swallow study and upper GI (UGI) series examines esophageal and stomach function and focuses on the anatomy of the esophagus, stomach, and duodenum. The barium swallow, completed by a radiologist, identifies mucosal and anatomical abnormalities, esophageal strictures, tumors, and esophageal motility. It has low sensitivity for diagnosing gastroesophageal reflux, which is better assessed with pH monitoring and/or manometry. This test is conducted with the patient positioned upright and in the supine position while swallowing liquid barium or, in some cases, a barium tablet. Since the esophagus is under involuntary neural control, compensatory swallowing strategies cannot be assessed with this procedure. However, recommendations can be made for changing to liquid consistencies in a patient with an esophageal stricture.

Esophagogastroduodenoscopy

In contrast, endoscopic evaluation of the entire UGI tract, or esophago-gastroduodenoscopy (EGD), is completed by a gastroenterologist and confirms the presence of strictures and mucosal anomalies, tumors, or bleeding. Endoscopy uses a thin, flexible tube (endoscope) to look at the lining of the esophagus, stomach, and upper small intestine (duodenum).

The assistance of a gastroenterologist may be required in cases requiring palliative dilation of the esophagus.

Esophageal Manometry

This procedure measures the strength and pattern of muscle contractions in the esophagus by the use of pressure readings. Lower esophageal sphincter (LES) muscle pressure can also be taken. This test, completed by a gastroenterologist, helps determine whether there is a problem with motility of the esophagus or the function of the LES.

pH Probe

An ambulatory 24-hour pH probe is a test that consists of a small tube passed through the nose into the esophagus. The tip of the tube has pH sensor that measures acid exposure in the esophagus and collects the data on a portable computer. These results are compared with "normal" acid exposure in the esophagus. This is considered the "gold standard" for determining the presence of gastroesophageal reflux disease (GERD).

Management of Dysphagia

Direct Swallowing Intervention

Active strengthening exercises and rehabilitation aimed at restoring or improving swallowing function may be recommended by the SLP following a swallowing assessment, although consideration of overall goals of care and treatment plan should be closely aligned. Exercises may be aimed at increasing tongue strength or movement, pharyngeal contraction, heightened airway and vocal fold closure, and increased opening of the UES. Like any other strengthening program, exercises are only beneficial in certain instances, such as when muscle strength is impaired and can be improved, and must be individualized to the specific dysfunction. The effectiveness and appropriateness of direct swallowing intervention in a patient with a degenerative process, or with advanced stages of disease may be questionable. Therefore, it will be necessary to discuss realistic impact and the appropriate implementation of a course of swallowing exercises. There are many causes of dysphagia other than muscle weakness, such as dementia-related cognitive impairment, that will not benefit from direct strengthening. Lastly, the overall level of endurance and cognitive ability to follow directions will also need to be considered before starting an exercise program.

Compensatory Swallowing Strategies

The physiologic information obtained from clinical and instrumental swallowing assessment facilitates determination of intervention strategies aimed at increasing swallowing safety and efficiency. These include alterations in head and neck posture, consistency of food, sensory awareness, and feeding behaviors. The principal advantage of these strategies is that they are simple for the patient to learn and to perform. In addition, once their effectiveness is determined, the patient can improve swallow function use during meals by utilizing these interventions. In 2008, a large, multisite, randomized clinical trial of patients with a diagnosis of dementia and/or PD was published examining the effects of three compensatory interventions to prevent aspiration of liquids, including chin-down posture, nectar-thickened liquids, and honey-thickened liquids. It demonstrated that strategies must be highly individualized, that there is no uniform effectiveness in any one of these strategies, and that effectiveness can only be determined by an objective swallowing evaluation.[8]

Postural Modifications

Postural changes during swallowing often have the effect of diverting the food or liquid to prevent aspiration or obstruction but do not change the swallowing physiology. A commonly used strategy is the chin-tuck posture. This posture has the advantage of increasing the pressure on the bolus and restricting the opening of the larynx during swallowing, thus potentially reducing the risk of laryngeal penetration and aspiration. However, in select cases, a chin tuck may exacerbate the aspiration, underscoring the need for radiographic evidence of its clinical value, if at all possible. These strategies may be used in isolation or in combination, depending on the nature of the underlying swallowing pathophysiology. Table 4.1 lists some of the postural strategies that the SLP may introduce, and their potential benefits on bolus flow.

Changes in Texture, Consistency, and Nutritional Content of Food

Changes in the consistency of food and liquid necessitate emotional adjustment and support for patients because they are often unappealing. Thus, this management strategy should be reserved for patients who are unable to follow directions to use postural changes or for whom other compensatory strategies are not feasible.[4] Underlying physiological impairments, such as reduced tongue control or strength, may affect the safety of swallowing certain food consistencies. Some patients may exhibit signs of aspiration on thin liquids, but may have sufficient control to drink liquids thickened to nectarlike or honeylike consistency in small sips. Patients debilitated by chronic disease and who lack endurance to complete a meal may benefit from ground or pureed moist foods that require limited mastication. In certain circumstances, the initiation of altered food consistency is the only option to assure a patient's comfort or safe oral intake. Examples and rationale of modified diets are listed in Table 4.2.

Specialized commercial agents derived from modified food starch or gum-based (xanthan, guar, cellulose) thickeners can be used to thicken liquids. Gum-based thickeners have improved performance over starch-based in terms of stability over time and temperature. Thickened liquids release the fluid in the gastrointestinal tract, do not alter the body's absorption rate of fluids, and provide water for hydration requirements. Additionally, some nutritional supplement drinks are thicker liquids and calorically fortified, providing a safer alternative to more solid consistencies, while others come in a pudding format.

The patient and caregivers should understand and consider the competing benefits and risks regarding nutrition, with attention to the patient's preferences. A guiding principle for the diet of an individual with dysphagia is to ingest the maximum amount of calories for the least amount of effort. A patient with dysphagia who requires adaptations in texture and

Table 4.1 Compensatory Postural Changes That Improve Bolus Flow and May Reduce Aspiration and Residue During Swallowing

Postural Strategy	Rationale
Chin tuck	Closes larynx, pushes tongue closer to posterior pharyngeal wall, and promotes epiglottic deflection
Head back	Promotes bolus movement through the oral cavity with assistance of gravity
Head tilt to stronger side	Directs bolus down stronger side with assistance of gravity
Head turned to weaker side	Diverts bolus away from weaker side of pharynx, promotes opening of upper esophagus
Head tilt plus chin tuck	Directs bolus down stronger side while increasing closure of larynx
Head rotation plus chin tuck	Diverts bolus away from weaker side while facilitating closure of laryngeal vestibule and vocal folds

Adapted from Logemann JA, Gensler G, Robbins J, et al. A randomized study of three interventions for aspiration of thin liquids in patients with dementia or Parkinson's disease. JSLHR. 2008;51(1):173–183.

Table 4.2 Diet Modifications for Patients With Dysphagia

Diet	Definition	Example	Indication
Pureed diet	Blenderized food with added liquid to form smooth consistency. No chewing necessary.	Applesauce, yogurt, moist mashed potatoes, puddings	Significantly reduced chewing, impaired pharyngeal contraction, esophageal stricture
Mechanically altered diet	Ground, finely chopped or diced foods that easily form a cohesive bolus with minimal chewing.	Pasta, soft scrambled eggs, cottage cheese, ground meats	Some limited chewing possible, but protracted
Soft, moist diet	Naturally soft foods requiring some chewing; food is cut in small pieces; serve with gravy to moisten.	Soft meats, canned fruits, baked fish. Avoid raw vegetables, bread, nuts, and tough meats	Reduced endurance for prolonged meal, reduced attention span; tongue/lip weakness
Liquids	Nectar consistency	Similar in viscosity to tomato juice; less thick than honey consistency	Reduced liquid bolus control, delayed swallow initiation and airway closure
	Honey consistency	Similar in viscosity to honey; available in ready-to-serve packaging or use thickening agent	Reduced oral or lingual control of liquid bolus, delayed swallow initiation and airway closure

consistency, or supplemental alternative nutrition, benefits from a collaborative approach to maximize safety, health, and satisfaction with eating.[9] Nutritionists can provide individualized suggestions for calorie-dense foods or high-calorie nutritional supplements, depending on the patient's metabolic status. Food preparation in a manner that increases caloric and nutritional value, as well as maximizing hydration is helpful. A close partnership and collaboration with the registered dietician (a specialist who performs a nutrition assessment and develops a nutrition care plan) will ensure the best outcome. Box 4.2 provides a list of cookbooks that can assist patients and care providers in preparing foods and liquids that have altered textures and may be easier to swallow.

Increased Sensory Awareness

Sensory enhancement techniques include increasing downward pressure of a spoon against the tongue when presenting food in the mouth and presenting a sour bolus, a cold bolus, a bolus requiring chewing, or a large-volume bolus. These techniques may elicit a quicker pharyngeal swallow response while reducing the risk of aspiration. Some patients benefit from receiving food or liquid at a slower rate, while others are more efficient with larger boluses. Enhancing the bolus characteristics to include more texture can sometimes induce mastication and bolus formation more readily than a bolus that is both flavorless and homogeneous in texture. This is particularly evident in patients with advanced dementia. Patient responses to these behaviors can be evaluated at the bedside, and the findings can be easily communicated to the caregivers.

Pharmacological and Medical Management of Dysphagia

There are no pharmacological agents that have been shown to directly act on oropharyngeal swallowing function. Studies on medical treatment such as hyperbaric oxygen therapy and medications that increase oxygenation or that may mediate the effects of fibrosis in head and neck cancer patients

---

Box 4.2 Cookbooks for Altered Food Consistency Diets

Gourmet Puree Recipes: The Ultimate Collection. Daniel Tyler. Amazon Digital Services, 2013.

Soft Foods for Easier Eating. Sandra Woodruff, MS, RD, LDN, and Leah Gilbert-Henderson, PhD, LDN. Square One Publishers, 2011.

Eat Well Stay Nourished: A Recipe and Resources Guide for Coping With Eating Challenges. Compiled and edited by Nancy E. Leupold. Published by SPOHNC, Support for People with Oral and Head and Neck Cancer, 2000.

Easy-to-Swallow, Easy-to-Chew Cookbook: Over 150 Tasty and Nutritious Recipes for People Who Have Difficulty Swallowing. Donna Weihoffen, JoAnne Robbins, Paula Sullivan. John Wiley, 2002.

The Dysphagia Cookbook. Elayne Achilles. Cumberland House, 2004.

I-Can't-Chew Cookbook. J. Randy Wilson and Mark A. Piper. Hunter House, 2003.

are inconclusive. However, there are agents for concurrent issues, which can exacerbate an underlying mucosal problem, and medications that may effectively treat the following:

- GI motility—prokinetic agents
- Reflux—proton pump inhibitors or histamine-2 blockers
- Nausea and vomiting—antiemetics
- Yeast infections such as candidiasis—topical nystatin, ketoconazole, miconazole, fluconazole, amphotericin B
- Sialorrhea (excess secretions)—botulinum toxin

Other Interventions

Complementary and Alternative Medicine

It is estimated that nearly half of all Americans practice some form of complementary and alternative medicine (CAM), and there is an increasing rise in interest in these treatments. Clinical evidence for CAM therapy for dysphagia and some of the underlying symptoms is somewhat limited for certain treatments. Acupuncture following stroke has raised much interest because dysphagia can be prevalent and debilitating in this population. However, two Cochrane reviews were unable to demonstrate clear evidence to support the use of acupuncture for dysphagia after stroke, and more large-scale trials are needed to determine its clinical efficacy.[10] Lastly, there are some promising results using acupuncture to treat GERD and esophageal dysmotility.

Oral Hygiene/Oral Care

The status of the oral mucosa and general oral hygiene reflect a patient's ability to manage secretions and swallowing. Oral health is often compromised in those who are critically ill, while oral hygiene can be neglected in tube-fed patients. A clean and moist oral cavity is not for patient comfort, but can reduce nosocomial infections and thereby reduce days in the hospital and other negative outcomes. Patients who require supplemental oxygen delivered via a nasal cannula frequently experience dryness in the oral cavity, which may further exacerbate, and in some cases even cause, difficulty swallowing. Severe illness and many medications may alter the normal oral environment, salivary production, and the growth of oral bacteria. This change in oral flora increases risk of bacterial pneumonia in critically ill patients as a result of aspiration of contaminated secretions. It is not uncommon to find dry secretions crusted along the tongue, palate, and pharynx in patients who have not eaten orally in some time. Dental caries and dentures that are not well cared for can also contribute to a state of poor oral hygiene as well as poor quality of life.

The American Association of Critical-Care Nurses issued a practice alert starting in 2006 for oral care procedures that include: frequent oral assessments, suctioning, and providing moisture to the lips and oral mucosa.[11] Other measures included the following:

- Prior to giving the patient food, liquids, or oral medications, it is vital to carefully inspect and assess the condition of the entire oral cavity with the use of a flashlight. Clear the oral cavity of extraneous secretions, using mouth swabs, tongue scrapers, toothbrushes, and oral suction if necessary.

- Providing humidification via a shovel mask or face tent and consistent oral care for the hospitalized patient may help to loosen secretions, moisten the oropharyngeal mucosa, and maximize comfort. Caution should be taken when completing oral care, as dried oral secretions may loosen during trials of fluid and inadvertently obstruct the airway.
- Chlorhexidine, a broad-spectrum antibacterial agent, is highly effective in reducing the risk of nosocomial respiratory infections and ventilator-associated pneumonia in critically ill patients.

Oral Feeding Options

Effortless, efficient, and safe swallowing are important criteria for continued oral nutrition. While there is no cure for a swallowing disorder in palliative care patient, continued oral intake may be facilitated by careful hand-feeding techniques employed by family and caregivers. These techniques will vary depending on the underlying swallowing/feeding difficulty. Hand feeding has been found to produce similar outcomes of death, aspiration pneumonia, functional status, and patient comfort for patients with dementia as initiating tube feeding. The respect for the ethical principle of patient autonomy within in a shared decision-making process is a critical. It should be accompanied by a clear understanding of the risks involved in oral intake. Specifically, families and patients should be informed about the risks and consequences of developing aspiration pneumonia and malnutrition. If the decision is to continue with oral intake, even if it impacts sufficient nutrition, the safest diet should be suggested and aspiration precautions introduced, using assessment of the swallowing problem as a guide. Family members are more likely to feed a patient a particular diet and in a particular manner if they understand the physiological and psychological reasons for the recommendation and if they have been included in the decision-making.

Additional suggestions for feeding the patient with dysphagia include:

1. *Remove distractions at mealtime.* This can help patients who need to concentrate on swallowing to increase safety, individuals who are using compensatory swallowing strategies, and patients who easily lose their focus and need to be fed, such as patients with dementia.
2. *Emphasize heightened awareness of sensory cues.* Feeding patients larger boluses and increasing downward pressure of the spoon on the tongue alert the patient that food is in the mouth. Feeding patients cold or sour boluses or foods requiring some mastication may improve oral sensation and awareness. Some patients with dementia demonstrate the most efficient swallow when offered finger foods that require chewing, allowing them greater access to the automatic motor rhythm of chewing and swallowing that is reminiscent of the patterns they have used all their lives.
3. *Provide feeding utensils.* Patients who have feeding difficulties associated with hand tremors or weakness may be aided with devices such as weighted cuffs or built-up utensils.

4. *Optimize the position of the patient.* Ensure optimal posture of the patient at meals. Sit the patient as upright as possible when eating, drinking, or taking medications. Reduce the tendency to slump forward or to the side, or to extend the head, which can promote an open airway and make the patient more vulnerable to aspiration.
5. *Schedule meal times.* Timing of meals to coincide with increased function, either due to effects from fatigue or medications may enhance swallowing efficiency and safety.
6. *Consider more frequent, smaller meals with high-calorie supplements.* Increased frequency of small meals may help patients who do not have sufficient efficiency or endurance to complete an entire meal at one time.

Medication Administration

Oral medications can present enormous challenges to patients with dysphagia. One study looking at pill swallowing in patients with chronic dysphagia found that more than 60% of subjects had difficulty swallowing tablets. Some of the physiologic difficulties they experienced included multiple swallows to clear the pill, residue in the pharynx after swallowing, increased time needed to swallow pills, use of liquid to assist in washing the pill down, and airway compromise. Because difficulty swallowing may impact compliance with medications, finding alternative modes of presentation can be critical.

Medications deemed nonessential may be temporarily or permanently discontinued. Crushing medications or burying them whole in a semisolid food such as applesauce or ice cream creates a uniform consistency and makes swallowing easier. However, crushing, opening, or chewing a medicine can alter its pharmacological properties, render it unlicensed, and may result in a potentially toxic and lethal dose.[12] Thus, always clarify whether a medication can be altered. Patients can be offered their medications in elixir form.

Consider alternative routes for medication administration including transdermal, buccal, or rectal.

Compounding, done by a pharmacist, creates a medication tailored to the specialized needs of an individual patient by producing an alternative form such as a powder, nebulized substances, liquid, lozenge, or suppository. However, compounded medications are not FDA approved, their safety and effectiveness are not verified, and most third-party payers at this time will not reimburse. Due to recent tragic events occurring as a result of nonsterile injectable medications, this practice is currently under scrutiny. Healthcare providers and patients should refer to the FDA statement on regulation of compounded drugs found at http://www.fda.gov/Drugs/GuidanceComplianceRegulatoryInformation/PharmacyCompounding/default.htm.

Orally disintegrating medication (ODT) technology has been used to formulate medications that rapidly disintegrate in the oral cavity once placed on or under the tongue. FDA guidelines regarding ODTs can be found at http://www.fda.gov/downloads/Drugs/GuidanceComplianceRegulatoryInformation/Guidances/UCM070578.pdf.

Alternative Nutrition and Hydration

For patients with a disease process that results in dysphagia and an inability to swallow, a decision may need to be made regarding placement of a gastrostomy or jejunostomy tubes to provide alternative hydration and nutrition. Expected medical benefits often include improved nutrition and hydration, easier administration of medications, prolongation of life, prevention of aspiration, diminished pain, and facilitation of nursing home placement. Irrespective of the scenario, the following should be considered:

1. Patients and their families need to be fully informed regarding benefits and risks of nonoral and oral feeding options in order to make fully informed decisions and to incorporate patient's wishes early into the care plan. For certain conditions, early placement of tube feeding may provide the patient with several more months of improved quality of life afforded by strength and endurance. Patients and families may also feel a sense of relief afforded to them because of the tube feeding itself.

2. However, a growing body of literature shows that overall there are limited medical benefits in improving survival rates, reducing aspiration risk, or improving functional status and that the expected benefits may exceed actual outcomes.[13]

3. The presence of a feeding tube does not inherently imply NPO, or nothing by mouth. Some patients may continue to take small amounts of food or liquid for their pleasure and comfort.

4. More creative solutions may help to ease the feeding decision. Although hand feeding is time consuming, it allows for continued intimate contact between patient and caregiver. One prominent geriatrician has proposed creating new solutions, such as Ensure lollipops or sublingual high-calorie drops.

Sialorrhea and Secretion Management

Sialorrhea, or excessive salivation and drooling due to the inability to control oral secretions, is common in patients with neurological conditions such as motor neuron disease and PD, with estimates of up to 80% of patients with PD experiencing excessive salivation. This is caused by:

- Impaired swallowing function
- Reduced frequency of swallowing
- Reduced oropharyngeal or laryngeal sensation
- Poor head posture
- Inability to close the oral cavity
- Weak cough with poor clearance of secretions

Hypersecretion may also occur in the setting of oral or dental infection, as a side effect of medication, or following extensive surgical reconstruction and repair such as in head and neck cancer. Excessive salivation can be embarrassing and socially disabling, as well as contribute to skin irritation, poor oral health, dehydration, and increased risk of aspiration pneumonia. In the early stages, behavioral, compensatory, and/or strengthening exercises via speech-language therapy to improve oromotor function and sensation, tongue control, self-management, and general body posture may be helpful.

In more severe disease, treatment options include anticholinergic medications (glycopyrrolate, scopolamine, benzotropine); botulinum toxin; radiation therapy to the parotid and submandibular glands; and surgical resection of either the parasympathetic neural pathway or of the submandibular and salivary glands. However, each of these treatment options has significant side effects, such as thickened secretions that are more difficult to expectorate, mucus plugging, dehydration, constipation, and drowsiness, and may be contraindicated or poorly tolerated in various populations.

Caregiver and Family Members' Experience

The experience of a family member providing care for a terminally ill patient is stressful. Managing the tube feeding, care of a gastrostomy tube stoma, changing diet textures, and altering social lives due to dysphagia is a significant burden, both physical and psychological. One study that examined the experience of caring for a dysphagic relative with head and neck cancer revealed the stress of becoming a "nurse—caregiver," the sense of "living between tube feedings" and feeling tied down by it, and the distress experienced from an inability to attend important social events because of the dysphagic individual's inability to eat. Partnering with the caregiver and the healthcare team's engagement with the caregiver throughout the care of the dysphagic patient at the end of- life is essential to alleviating burden and stress to the extent possible.

Dry Mouth (Xerostomia)

Definition

Xerostomia is the sensation of oral dryness, which may or may not be accompanied by decreased salivary secretions. Xerostomia is also known as salivary gland dysfunction or hyposalivation.[14] Although patients receiving palliative care commonly experience oral dryness, it is often difficult to identify the exact underlying cause and/or contributing factors.[15] Decreased salivary function and prolonged xerostomia cause significant oral symptoms in the mouth, including:

- Dental caries
- Oral pain
- Gum, tongue, and oral mucosal irritations and lesions
- Mouth infections
- Taste changes and bad breath
- Swallowing difficulties
- Alterations in speech formation and voice function
- Physical discomfort
- Emotional suffering
- Retreat from socializing[16]

In several studies, xerostomia appears to be common in 30%–50% of patients.[17] Other authors estimate that xerostomia affects 30% of palliative care patients. In palliative care, xerostomia appears to be a major source of discomfort in patients with cancer. Well described in the cancer literature, it has been described in other conditions: diabetes, end-stage renal failure, end-stage cardiac disease, and end-stage liver disease. In the population at large, xerostomia increases with age and medical problems because medication therapy increases.

Pathophysiology

Dry mouth is rooted in reduced saliva. Saliva is produced by numerous glands in the oropharynx. The average production of saliva in a healthy adult is 1.5 liters a day. The parotid glands, the submandibular glands, and the sublingual glands produce 90% of saliva, the other 10% is produced in the oral pharynx. Parotid glands, located below and in front of each ear, produce a serous and watery saliva. Therefore, damage to the parotid gland will produce a thicker saliva. Submandibular glands, located in the lower jaw, secrete mostly serous saliva with some mucinous elements. Sublingual glands produce purely mucous saliva. The overall viscosity of saliva is dependent on the functioning of the various glands.

Saliva is necessary to the process of oral nutrition in initiating the breakdown of food; it also facilitates chewing, swallowing, and talking. The properties of saliva allow oral lubrication and gum and tissue repair and help in gustation with food-bolus formation and food breakdown. Additionally, saliva breaks down bacterial substances, offering immunoprotection for oral mucosa and dental structures. Saliva thereby inhibits dental caries and infections, while providing protection against extreme temperatures of food and drink.[18] Saliva production is regulated by the nervous system. Within 2 to 3 seconds, smell, sight, or taste of food stimulates salivary production. There is a two-step process to saliva secretion: (1) production at the acinar level of the cells and (2) secretion, where saliva is actually secreted into the mouth via the ducts. Saliva comprises several elements. Ninety-nine percent of saliva is fluid composed of water and mucus, providing a lubricative element. The remaining 1% of saliva is solid, containing salts, proteins, minerals such as calcium bicarbonate ions, and enzymes such as pytalin, antibodies, and other antimicrobial agents. Four general categories of xerostomia exist:

1. Reduced salivary secretions
2. Buccal erosion
3. Local or systemic dehydration
4. Other miscellaneous conditions

Reduced salivary secretion is commonly caused by medication side effects, infections, hypothyroidism, autoimmune processes, and sarcoidosis. Oral dryness may result from oral diseases such as acute and chronic parotitis, or partial or complete salivary obstruction. In cancer patients, reduced saliva production may be caused by tumor-induced salivary gland destruction or treatment. Cancer treatment, including both radiation and chemotherapy, affects salivary production. Radiation to the head and neck can reduce saliva production by 50% to 60% within the first week of treatment because of inflammation. Chemotherapy and cytotoxic agents may also cause dry mouth, particularly in advanced disease. Medications are notorious culprits of dry mouth, particularly several classifications common in of medications commonly used in palliative care: sedatives, tranquilizers, antihistamines, antiparkinsonian medications, antiseizure medications, skeletal muscle relaxants, tricyclic antidepressants, and anticholinergics.

Buccal erosion frequently occurs in cancer and cancer treatment, particularly chemotherapy and radiation. The duration of radiation and/or radiation doses affects the persistence and degree of salivary reduction. In addition, buccal erosion and subsequent dry mouth is common in immune-related conditions such as Sjögren's syndrome, diabetes mellitus, HIV/AIDS, scleroderma, sarcoidosis, lupus, Alzheimer's disease, and graft versus host disease.

Systemic dehydration-induced xerostomia results from a wide spectrum of conditions including debility, anorexia, vomiting, diarrhea, fever, drying oxygen therapies, mouth breathing, polyuria, diabetes, hemorrhage, and swallowing difficulties. Mental health issues may induce dry mouth including depression, coping reactions, anxiety, and depression. Due to diurnal production, dry mouth sensations are worse at night, resulting in sleep interruptions. Over longer periods of time, lack of sleep may cause anxiety, depression, and distress as part of the stress response.

The number of comorbidities with resultant complex pharmacotherapy, and not the age of the patient, increases the risk of xerostomia.[19] These same comorbidities make the management of plaque and gums difficult. Patients undergoing cancer treatment or other immunosuppressive therapies may be too immunocompromised to undergo oral surgery or treatment procedures. Thus, patients may experience simultaneous discomfort from their chronic progressive illness, or serious life-threatening illness as well as subsequent oral distress.

Assessment

As stated above, xerostomia is a dry mouth. However, it may be accompanied by other oral symptoms such as burning, smarting, and soreness of both the oral mucosa and the tongue, with or without the presence of ulcers. There may be difficulty with mastication, swallowing, and speech. Or, there may be taste alterations, difficulty with dentures, and an increase in dental caries subsequent to the lack of the protective characteristics of saliva. Common secondary concerns are nutritional issues, sleep, and rest.[20,21] Therefore, a thorough history should review these problem areas along with the subjective distress of xerostomia and current medications.[22]

A thorough assessment will assist in determining etiology. Assessment should include patient rating in eight aspects of dry mouth. These areas include overall mouth and lip dryness, speech, chewing, sleeping, dry mouth with eating and swallowing, resting, and the frequency of sipping liquids for eating and during the rest of the day. Sample questions are included in Box 4.3.

Oral Examination

An intraoral examination will reveal clear indications of dry mouth: pale and dry mucosal and buccal areas, the presence of a dry and fissured tongue, a red raw tongue, the absence of salivary pooling, and the presence of oral ulcerations, gingivitis, or candidiasis. Salivary glands should be noted for

Box 4.3 Xerostomia Assessment Questions[19,21,22]

Do you experience dry mouth? How frequently?

Does dry mouth bother you?

Do you have dry lips?

Do you have dry nasal passages?

Do your gums bleed when you brush your teeth?

Is your tongue red and raw?

Do you find there are times you need to drink more fluids? When?

Do you experience difficulty speaking due to a dry or sticky mouth?

Do you have difficulty chewing? What types of foods?

Do you have difficulty swallowing? Solids or liquids?

Do you need extra fluid to help you swallow food? All foods or solids or semisolids?

Do you use hard candies or gum for your dry mouth?

Do you find your sleep is disrupted by dry mouth? How often do you wake up at night because of a dry mouth?

Have you experienced altered taste sensations? What types of tastes? Any types of foods?

Do you use tobacco? How often?

Do you drink alcohol? How often?

Do you drink caffeine? In what drinks? In what foods?

Are you taking any prescription medications or over-the-counter medications or preparations?

swelling, indicating obstruction, and dentition should be examined for caries. Extraoral examination reveals cracked lips, often with angular cheilitis (lip inflammation) or candida at the corners of the mouth.

There are several diagnostic tests for xerostomia, saliva measurement, and dry mouth evaluation. There are two standard bedside tests for xerostomia: the cracker biscuit test and the tongue blade test.

- The cracker biscuit test involves giving a patient a dry cracker or biscuit. If the patient cannot eat the cracker without extra fluids, xerostomia is present.

- The tongue blade test is an extension of mouth inspection. After inspection is complete, the tongue blade is placed on the tongue. Since dry mouth makes for ropey, pasty saliva, the tongue blade will stick to the tongue of a patient with xerostomia.

- Another, more aggressive test is unstimulated or stimulated sialometric measurement of saliva. This test measures the amount of saliva collected by spitting into a container, swabbing the mouth with a cotton-tipped applicator, or salivating into a test container at a set time. However, for most palliative care patients, this may be a burdensome and unnecessary test.

Documentation of the extent of xerostomia is essential. There are many rating scales specifically designed for this purpose. There are several scales suggested in Box 4.4. The American Dental Hygienists' documentation is the most comprehensive, versus documentation based only on saliva changes as offered by the American Cancer Society or the Oncology Nursing Society.

Prevention

Prevention occurs in pretreatment considerations. The National Institute of Dental and Craniofacial Research suggests a pretreatment screening ideally 4 to 6 weeks prior to the commencement of any treatments. During this screening assessment, oral examination is performed to identify potential issues, such as infection, fractured teeth or restorations, or periodontal disease that could contribute to oral complications once treatment begins. The evaluation also establishes baseline data for comparison in subsequent examinations. Should any treatment such as fillings, extractions, or periodontal surgery be necessary before treatment initiation, 2 weeks of recovery allows time for healing and reduces further complications of infection from low blood counts. Further education about both the importance and comfort of good oral care is essential.

Management

Much of xerostomia management focuses on interventions to alleviate rather than interventions to eradicate or to prevent the symptom. The goal is to protect patients from further complications. A stepwise approach should guide management and treatment, as suggested in Box 4.5. Table 4.3 offers suggestions for pharmacological management.[14,22]

Box 4.4 Dry Mouth Rating Scales

American Dental Hygienists Association[19]

Tissue changes (tongue and mucosal color)
Oral disease (bad breath, cavities, infection)
Saliva, glands, and function

American Cancer Society Radiation Side Effects—Dry Mouth[23]

Decreased saliva
Thick saliva
No saliva

Oncology Nursing Society Xerostomia[24]

0 No dry mouth
1 Mild dryness, slightly thickened saliva, little change in taste
2 Moderate dryness, thick and sticky saliva, markedly altered taste
3 Complete dryness of mouth
4 Salivary necrosis

Box 4.5 Stepwise Process for Managing Xerostomia[22]

1. Treat underlying infections—Candidiasis should be treated using nystatin swish-and-swallow or fluconazole 150 mg PO.

2. Review and alter current medications as appropriate. It is important to first evaluate the necessity of specific xerostomia-inducing drugs. There are numerous medications that list oral dryness as a side effect. Specifically, anticholinergics, antihistamines, phenothiazines, antidepressants, opioids, beta blockers, diuretics, anticonvulsants, sedatives, and tobacco all may cause oral dryness. Thus, patients with heart conditions, mental health issues, depression, anxiety, neurological disorders, and pain disorders may be at risk for dry mouth. If eliminating possible culprit medication is not possible, other possible strategies include decreasing the dosage to decrease dryness, or altering the schedule to assure that the peak effect of medication does not coincide with nighttime peak of decreased salivary production.

3. Stimulate salivary flow—Salivary stimulation can occur with both nonpharmacological and pharmacological interventions.

4. Replace lost secretions with saliva substitutes—Saliva substitutes are better tolerated than artificial salivas. Oral spray preparations are best tolerated. Saliva substitutes are based on aqueous solution and may contain carboxymethyl cellulose or mucin from animals. Attention must be paid to any philosophical, cultural, or religious prohibitions concerning the animal ingredients of saliva substitutes.

5. Protect teeth—Continue meticulous mouth care. Protect with fluoride rinses.

6. Rehydrate—Drink plenty of liquids.

7. Modify diet—to avoid mouth pain from acids or hard foods.

Nonpharmacological Interventions

Nonpharmacological interventions should be tried first. Of course preventive measures may help reduce dry mouth. Nonpharmacological use of gustatory stimulation includes a myriad of measures (see Table 4.4).[14,22,25] All of these interventions are short term and relatively inexpensive with few adverse effects. Insurances may cover some of these costs as well except procedures. Acupuncture during and after radiation therapy for head and neck cancer has been found to prevent chronic dry mouth. A randomized controlled trial using acupuncture concurrently with radiation therapy for patients with nasopharyngeal cancer reduced the incidence and severity of xerostomia and improved quality of life,[26] while another small sample study demonstrated that 9 of 10 patients treated with acupuncture for radiation-induced dysphagia and xerostomia reported subjective improvements in swallowing, xerostomia, and pain. Others have shown lasting benefits and effectiveness in other patient populations with xerostomia, such as Sjögren's syndrome, and recommend a 3- to 4-week regimen of weekly acupuncture treatments.

Table 4.3 Pharmacological Interventions

Medication	Description	Dose	Side Effect
Pilocarpine	Nonselective muscarinic A parasympathetic agent that increases exocrine gland secretion and stimulates residual functioning tissue in damaged salivary glands. Increases saliva production. New studies have shown that pilocarpine given before and during radiotherapy can reduce xerostomia.	Dose may be given at 5 mg TID or QID depending on how well patients tolerate the medication and its side effect.	Response varies with severity of xerostomia. Pilocarpine should not be used in patients with chronic obstructive pulmonary disease, asthma, bradycardia, renal or hepatic impairment, glaucoma, or bowel obstruction. Side effects include mild to moderate sweating, visual disturbances, nausea, rhinitis, chills, flushing, sweating, dizziness, increased urinary frequency, abdominal cramping, and asthenia. Side effects can be lessened if taken with milk.
Bethanechol	M-3 muscarinic relieves anticholinergic side effects of tricyclic antidepressants.		
Methacholine	A parasympathomimetic compound that increases salivation.	Dose is 10 mg a day.	Hypotension It is short acting.
Yohimbine	Blocks alpha-2 adrenoreceptors	Dose is 14 mg a day.	Drowsiness, confusion, and atrial fibrillation, lasting up to 3 hours.
Cevimeline	M-1 and M-3 muscarinic agonist. Acts to increase saliva by inhibiting acetylcholinesterase. Works on salivary glands and lacrimal glands, promoting increased salivary flow and tears in the eyes.	Used in a spray or mouthwash gargle, it lasts up to 6 hours.	Less effect than pilocarpine.

(continued)

Table 4.3 (Continued)

Medication	Description	Dose	Side Effect
Antifungals	May be needed for oral dryness caused by oral candidial infections.	First-line treatment is nystatin (suspension or troches, depending on swallowing ability), which is inexpensive. Second treatment includes fluconazole. Fungal infections of the lips may necessitate the use of miconazole, clotrimazole, or ketonacozole.	Taste changes

Table 4.4 Interventions for Xerostomia Management

Intervention	Role/Effect	Benefit	Comment
I. Preventative			
Oral Care	Reduces xerostomia severity. Promotes well-being		Frequent brushing with soft brushes, water jet, denture cleaning, fluoride rinses, mouthwash, and flossing, can stimulate salivation. This can help prevent candidiasis, particularly as dentures can harbor infections.
Lip Protectants	Prevents cracked lips and use of saliva to moisten lips. Includes use of lip protectants such as balms, chap sticks, and other preparations		Care should be taken not to use products with alcohol, as these can be irritating. Angular cheilitis at corners of the mouth requires protection with the use of lanolin and KY Jelly.
Dentifrices			Several are manufactured for patients with dry mouth that contain antimicrobial enzymes to reduce oral infections and enhance mouth wetting. Examples are Biotene, Oral Balance, and Oasis.
Mouthwashes Non-alcohol containing	Helps rinse debris from mouth.		Includes homemade mouthwashes made from saline, sodium bicarbonate, glycerin.

(continued)

Table 4.4 (Continued)

Intervention	Role/Effect	Benefit	Comment
II. Diet Modifications			
	Allows patient to eat.	Soft texture foods are better tolerated than rough foods. In addition, instruct patients to take fluids with all meals and snacks. The use of gravies and juices with foods can add moisture to swallowing.	Soups, pudding, mashed potatoes, and shakes rather than foods with rough edges such as crackers or toast. Olive oil or another light oil to the gums and mucosa may help act as a lubricant. Patients may sip such foods in milk, tea, or water to assist in swallowing. Education regarding the avoidance of sugars, spicy foods, sometimes salt, and dry or piquant foods is important, although preferred tastes may vary from one patient to the next. For dry mouth without oral ulcerations, provide carbonated drinks such as ginger ale, as well as cider, apple juice, or lemonade. Fresh fruits, papaya juice, or pineapple juice may help some patients refresh their mouths; however, citrus products may be too acidic and irritating for other patients.
III. Nonpharmacological			
Peppermint water	Mucous saliva	Inexpensive	Interacts with metoclopramide
Vitamin C	Chemical reduction Disrupts salivary mucin to reduce viscosity of saliva	Inexpensive Reduces viscosity	Can irritate mouth if sores present Use in lozenges or other forms as preferred. May be irritating to the mouth, particularly if the patient has mouth sores. Can erode dental enamel.
Citric acid/ sweets	For mucous saliva	Inexpensive	Can irritate, like vitamin C. In sweets, can cause caries. Presents in malic acid or in sweets. Can cause burning.

(continued)

Table 4.4 (Continued)

Intervention	Role/Effect	Benefit	Comment
Chewing gum, mints	For watery saliva. May create a buffer system to compensate for dietary acids. Effective as salivary stimulants due to the effect on chemoreceptors and mechanical receptors.	Inexpensive	Chewing gum is more effective than mints. In particular, a low tack gum is preferable for patients with dentures. Preferably, gum is sugarless, to prevent caries and infections, because an immunocompromised state promotes cavities and infections. Attention must be paid to social acceptance of gum chewing, particularly in older populations. Side effect of diarrhea from sorbitol if too much gum or mints taken.
Rehydration	Replenish oral hydration by sipping water, spraying water, and increasing humidity in the air		This includes adding humidity to oxygen systems, and using vaporizers to add humidity to counteract the drying effects of indoor heating and air conditioning. To assist in sleep, instituting these measures at night may help rest.
Saliva Replacement			
Water sprays or sip	Reduces pain or decreases saliva It is usually well tolerated and easily accessible	Inexpensive	Short acting There is no research on whether optimal relief results from either warm or cold. Thus, temperature is a personal choice.
Artificial saliva	Artificial saliva contains carboxy-methylcellulose or mucin; dose 2 mL every 3 to 4 hours.	Inexpensive	Those with a mucin base appear to be better tolerated than those derived from carboxymethylcellulose. Both types of preparation bases are better tolerated as an oral spray than as a gel or rinse.
Procedures			
Laser Treatment	Stimulate saliva production	Longer lasting Expensive	Administered in an office to salivary glands.

(continued)

Table 4.4 (Continued)

Intervention	Role/Effect	Benefit	Comment
Electro-stimulation	Stimulate saliva production	Longer lasting Less expensive than laser therapy	Delivered to the glands and tongue via a battery operated process.
Acupuncture	Increase production	Noninvasive Variable Costs	Can be expensive. Relief may occur in a single treatment or regular weekly treatment with needle placement in the ears and finger. One study showed that 6 weeks of twice-weekly treatment increased salivation for up to 1 year. Another study used a 3-to-4 weekly regimen, with monthly maintenance visits to relieve xerostomia.

Special Considerations for Older Adults With Impaired Cognition

There are several considerations to managing xerostomia in the patient with cognitive impairment. First, if a patient forgets oral care, the nurse should strategize on reminders and enlist family or other providers to assist. Second, their dentures need to be attended to and need to be thoroughly cleaned daily by brushing with appropriate cleansers. If the nurse is unable to remove or insert dentures to do oral exam due to the patient's agitation, the nurse may need another person to do simultaneous distraction or enlist the assistance of another provider while cleaning dentures. Third, if the patient refuses oral care, the nurse needs to assess the reason for refusal and ameliorate that issue if possible. If the patient bites on the toothbrush, have several available to allow the patient to bite on one while care occurs with another. Finally, if the patient has difficulty with mouthwash and toothpastes, it may be helpful for the nurse to use a suction toothbrush.

Nursing Interventions

Interventions will vary from one patient to the next based on the degree of xerostomia. Strong evidence supporting the efficacy of one treatment over another has not been demonstrated. Education is indispensable in dry mouth, and nurses provide essential information about xerostomia. During palliative treatments, patients need encouragement and support in ongoing dental care. This includes the use of soft toothbrushes, wetting the brush before using, the long-term need for fluoride rinses and toothpaste, and dietary restrictions of sugar to prevent further infections and caries. As a patient declines, teaching the family how to provide mouth care offers a tangible and important role in the comfort of the patient. Standardized oral care procedures and protocols vary from one institution to another. The nurse may help a family systematically trial a variety of therapies from nonpharmacological to pharmacological to achieve relief. However, goals of care and medication interactions and side effects should be reviewed in the context of the patient's overall condition.

Summary

As a symptom, dry mouth may be considered inconsequential. However, it has considerable quality-of-life implications. To create a suitable management plan, the nurse must assess the distress from xerostomia and determine financial considerations. Patients may be responsible to pay out-of-pocket costs for nonpharmacological interventions or may have limited coverage of pharmacological agents. Oral care and education are an essential strategy and may prevent severe dry mouth. There is no strong data to support pharmacological over nonpharmacological strategies. Patients may choose nonpharmacological therapy because it is inexpensive and has fewer side effects. Families will need to help manage the symptom as the patient declines. However, continued oral care can promote dignity.

Hiccups

Definition

Hiccup, or singultus, is defined as sudden, involuntary contractions of one or both sides of the diaphragm and intercostal muscles, terminated by an abrupt closure of the glottis, producing a characteristic sound of "hic." Hiccup occurs with a frequency of around 4 to 60 times per minute.[27] Prolonged hiccups result in fatigue and exhaustion from both respiratory insufficiency and sleep interferences. Anxiety, depression, and frustration result if eating and/or sleeping are routinely interrupted. Although seemingly insignificant, hiccups affect quality of life.

Prevalence and Impact

Hiccups in the palliative care population have undergone more review. However, the literature focuses on case studies rather than research into treatment. Therefore, the incidence and prevalence are not known. Prevalence of hiccups in cancer patients is estimated at 10% to 20%.

Pathophysiology

The precise pathophysiology and the physiological function of hiccups are not well understood. They are believed to be a primitive function, such as yawning or vomiting, that developed within the evolutionary process and now serves no discrete purpose. However, functionally, hiccups arise from a synchronous clonic spasm or spasmodic contraction of the diaphragm and the intercostal muscles, which results in sudden inspiration and prompt closure of the glottis, causing the hiccup sounds. The anatomical cause of hiccups is thought to be bimodal, with association either with the phrenic or vagus nerve, or central nervous involvement, which causes misfiring. It is hypothesized that a hiccup reflex arc is located within the phrenic nerves, the vagal nerves, and T6–T12 sympathetic fibers, as well as a possible hiccup center in either the respiratory center, the brainstem, or the cervical cord between C3 and C5. However, there does not appear to be a discrete hiccup center comparable to the chemoreceptor trigger zone for nausea.

Evidence suggests an inverse relationship between partial pressure of carbon dioxide (pCO_2) and hiccups; that is, an increased pCO_2 decreases the frequency of hiccups and a decreased pCO_2 increases frequency of hiccups. Interestingly, hiccups have a minimal effect on respiration, although they cause fatigue and a sensation of inability to take deep breaths. Hiccup strength or amplitude varies within discrete hiccup episodes as well as from patient to patient. This amplitude produces the distress, as continuous strong hiccups are exhausting because of the energy used in hiccupping.

There are three categories of hiccups: benign, persistent, and intractable hiccups.

- Benign, self-limiting hiccups occur frequently; an episode can last from several minutes to 2 days. The primary etiology is gastric distention; other causes include sudden changes in temperature, alcohol ingestion, excess smoking, and psychogenic alternations.

- Persistent, or chronic, hiccups continue for more than 48 hours but less than 1 month.

- Intractable hiccups persist longer than 1 month.[28,29] In palliative care, the duration may not be as important as the amplitude or strength of the hiccup depending on the population. For instance, a patient with ALS or COPD may have more distress than a cardiac patient, as they are already weak and breathing is compromised. Intractable hiccups result from more than 100 different causes ranging from metabolic disturbances to complex structural lesions of the CNS or infections.[27]

Particular causes can be consolidated into four categories: structural, metabolic, inflammatory, and infectious disorders.[27] Structural conditions specifically affect or irritate the peripheral branches of the phrenic and vagus nerves, such as in abdominal or mediastinal tumors, hepatomegaly, ascites, or gastric distention, and CNS disorders. Persistent hiccups can indicate serious underlying disorders, such as thoracic aneurysm, brainstem tumors, metabolic and drug-related disorders, infectious diseases, and psychogenic disorders.[27]

Common causes in terminal illness include neurological disorders such as stroke, brain tumors, and sepsis and metabolic imbalances; phrenic nerve irritations such as tumor compression or metastases; pericarditis, pneumonia, or pleuritis; and vagal nerve irritations such as esophagitis, gastric distention, gastritis, pancreatitis, hepatitis, and myocardial infarction.[27] Medications including steroids, chemotherapy, dopamine antagonists, megestrol, methyldopa, nicotine, opioids, and muscle relaxants may also cause hiccups. Dexamethasone, a frequently used palliative medication, may cause hiccups.[27]

Assessment

Extensive workup for hiccups in palliative care is impractical and uncomfortable and reveals little to assist in determining the etiology or delineating treatment. Studies have not revealed that laboratory tests provide any useful information to determine optimal management.[28] Nonetheless, assessment should include a subjective review of the qualitative distress induced by the hiccups. For example, in a patient with an abdominal or lung tumor, hiccups can cause excruciating pain, whereas in the obtunded patient in renal failure, hiccups may cause little distress at all.

In reviewing distress, it is important to evaluate conditions caused by the hiccups:

- Weight loss due to anorexia
- Fatigue due to the energy use from hiccups
- Inability to eat from impaired swallowing
- Shortness of breath from inability to take deep breaths
- Insomnia from hiccuping all night
- Heartburn from acid reflux produced by hiccups
- Depression resulting from all of the above

Objective assessment includes the history and duration of the current episode of hiccups, previous episodes, and interference with rest, eating, or daily routines.

- Inquiry into possible triggers may be helpful, including patterns during the day, and activities preceding the hiccups such as eating, drinking, or positioning.
- A review of recent trauma, surgery, procedures, and acute illness, as well as a medication history, is important to help focus on potential causes.

Further physical exam may not reveal much related to the hiccups themselves but rather assists in ruling out other conditions.

- Oral examination may reveal signs of swelling or obstruction.
- Observation of the patient's general appearance includes inspection for signs of a toxic or septic process. Any wounds or infections should be examined along with a thorough respiratory examination.
- More specifically, evaluation includes temporal artery tenderness, foreign bodies in the ear, infection of the throat, goiter in the neck, pneumonia or pericarditis of the chest, abdominal distention or ascites, and signs of stroke or delirium—all diagnoses that may have hiccups as part of the constellation of signs and symptoms.
- Abdominal distention, hepatomegaly, should be noted.

In very rare circumstances, specific testing may be warranted to eliminate other causes. Chest X-ray may rule out pulmonary or mediastinal processes, as well as phrenic/vagal irritation from peritumor edema in the abdominal area. Blood work including a complete blood count with differential electrolytes may rule out infection, as well as electrolyte imbalances and renal failure. Sometimes a CT scan of the abdomen or head may be done to rule out abnormalities or a cerebral bleed.

Management

The absence of larger randomized controlled studies on the nature of hiccups therapy has resulted in lack of consensus around treatment and anecdotal therapy.[28] Consequently, treatment is based on the bias of previous success rather than a systematic, evidence-based approach. Similar to treatment of dysphagia or xerostomia, treatment for hiccups should be focused on the underlying disease. If the etiology likely includes simple causes such as gastric distention or temperature changes, "empiric" treatment should be initiated. Both nonpharmacological and pharmacological interventions may be used.[28] Therapies include physical maneuvers, medications, and other procedures that interfere with the hiccup arc.[28] Otherwise, treatment for more complex episodes of hiccups without clear etiology will focus on various pharmacological interventions.

Nonpharmacological Treatment

Nonpharmacological treatments can be divided into seven categories and are outlined in Box 4.6.[22,27]

Box 4.6 Nonpharmacological Interventions for Hiccups[22,27]

Respiratory Measures

Breath holding

Rebreathing in a paper bag

Diaphragm compression

Ice application in mouth

Induction of sneeze or cough with spices or inhalants

Nasal and Pharyngeal Stimulation

Nose pressure

Stimulant inhalation

Tongue traction

Drinking from far side of glass

Swallowing sugar

Eating soft bread

Soft touch to palate with cotton-tipped applicator

Lemon wedge with bitters

Miscellaneous Vagal Stimulation

Ocular compression

Digital rectal massage

Carotid massage

Psychiatric Treatments

Behavioral techniques

Distraction

(Continued)

Box 4.6 (Continued)

Gastric Distention Relief

Fasting
Nasogastric tube to relieve abdominal distention
Lavage
Induction of vomiting

Phrenic Nerve Disruption

Anesthetic block
Phrenic block
Suboccipital release gentle traction and pressure applied to the posterior neck

Miscellaneous Treatments

Bilateral radial artery compression
Peppermint water to relax lower esophagus
Acupuncture

Pharmacological Treatment

Initial therapy should attempt to decrease gastric distention, the common cause in 95% of cases. Subsequent measures include hastening gastric emptying and relaxing the diaphragm with simethicone and metoclopramide. If ineffective, second-line therapy should focus on suppression of the hiccup reflex. Common pharmacological interventions are listed in Table 4.5.[22,27–29]

Nursing Interventions

Although hiccups appear to be a simple reflex, their specific mechanism of action is unclear, due to myriad etiologies. Many patients are frustrated because their discomfort and disruption were not taken seriously. The nurse can help discuss with the patient their concerns about treatment and their desire for comfort. Nursing interventions should focus on information regarding the broad range of strategies to eliminate the hiccups. Thus, the nursing role is one of advocate to promote comfort, empathetic listener, and educator.

The extent of aggressive treatment will depend on the degree of distress of the hiccups and the interference with quality of life—in particular, the extent of impact that hiccups have on the daily routine, specifically on sleep and nutrition. Information should include nonpharmacological maneuvers such as respiratory maneuvers, nasal and pharyngeal stimulation, distraction, and peppermint waters. If these measures fail to eradicate the hiccups, the nurse can discuss the range of pharmacological options and offer reassurance to continue various efforts because patients respond differently. Antacids may decrease gas, antiemetics may affect dopamine levels,

Table 4.5 Suggested Pharmacological Treatment for Hiccups

Agent	Effect
Agents to decrease gastric distention	
Simethicone 15–30 mL PO q 4 h	Promotes emptying
Metoclopramide 10–20 mg PO/IV q 4–6 h (cannot use with peppermint water)	Promotes gastric emptying
Muscle relaxants	
Baclofen 5–20 mg PO q 6–12 h up to 15–37 mg/d	Acts at synaptic level
Midazolam 5–10 mg PO q 4 h	Reduces muscles spasm
Anticonvulsants	
Gabapentin 300–600 mg PO TID	Acts on cortex area
Pregabalin 25 mg BID Pregabalin is active at lower doses and does not require a long titration (maximal doses can be reached within 1–2 weeks)	Interaction of pregabalin with the alpha-2 delta subunit inhibits N- and P/Q-type voltage-sensitive Ca^{2+} channels, which control neurotransmitter release in the brain and spinal cord
Carbamazepine 600–1200 mg PO QID-TID	Reduces muscle spasm
Valproic acid 15 mg/kg/24 h PO divided in one or three doses. May increase by 250 mg/wk until hiccups stop	Reduces muscle spasm
Phenytoin 200 mg IV × 1, then 100 mg PO QID	Reduces muscle spasm
Antidepressants	
Amitriptyline 10–50 mg PO	Acts at central nervous system
Sertraline 50–150 mg PO QD	Acts at central nervous system
Corticosteroids	
Dexamethasone 40 mg PO QD	Reduces inflammation
Dopamine agonists	
Haloperidol 2–10 mg PO/IV/SQ q 4–12 h	Reduces muscle spasm
Chlorpromazine 5–50 mg PO/IM/IV q 4–8 h or 25–50 mg IM/IV in 1 L 0.9% normal saline	Blocks dopamine and alpha-adrenergic receptors
Calcium channel blockers	
Lidocaine 1 mg/kg loading dose followed by infusion of 2 mg/min	Blocks sodium channels
Nifedipine 10–80 mg PO QD	Causes vasodilation to suppress spasm
Other medications	
Ketamine 0.4 mg/kg	Acts on cortex and limbic system
Amitriptyline 25–90 mg PO QD	Inhibits serotonin and norepinephrine uptake

and muscle relaxants may affect both gamma-aminobutyric acid channels and skeletal muscle. Separately they may be ineffective, but together they target several regions that trigger hiccups.

If all of these medications fail to induce hiccup reduction or cessation, the nurse should suggest a referral to a palliative care service, a pain service, or an anesthesia service to explore further treatment options. These services can consider possible invasive procedures such a nerve block, or infusion. However, as always, discussion with the patient should include prognosis and the benefit and burden of any procedure. If hiccups become extremely burdensome and all therapies have failed, sedation may be a consideration. Again, the nurse may act as an advocate to provide the necessary information about the implications of sedation.

Summary

The development of hiccups can truly affect quality of life. Though perceived as more of an annoyance rather than a symptom, hiccups can impact sleep, rest, speech, and oral nutrition. The challenge is that there is not clear evidence of one treatment over another. Quality of life and goals of care should dictate management, particularly as medications have significant side effects that may be unacceptable to the patient. Expert consensus suggests a systematic approach of nonpharmacological interventions should be initiated by pharmacological interventions. It is hoped that more research into hiccups will offer evidence-based practice.

Conclusion

Dysphagia, xerostomia, and hiccups are common problems that have not garnered much interest in research. There is more research to support evidence-based practice for dysphagia management. A multidisciplinary approach utilizing nurses, SLPs, nutritionists, dietitians, and social workers will promote successful treatment. On the other hand, xerostomia and hiccups are considered minor symptoms. Therefore, they appear to be underreported and underestimated. Nurses at the bedside, whether in a facility or at home, may be the first to identify the presence of these symptoms and understand the negative impact on quality of life. The mere act of listening to a patient's distress offers affirmation of the existence of the symptoms and validation that the symptoms will be taken seriously. Given the lack of hard evidence to manage these symptoms, the nurse must be creative in his or her approach. Working with a team can offer relief to patients and their families.

Acknowledgment

The authors would like to acknowledge and thank Tessa Goldsmith, MS, CCC-SLP, who served as the original coauthor of this chapter in the first edition and third author in the second edition of the *Oxford Textbook of*

Palliative Nursing, for the excellent foundation of the dysphagia portion of this chapter.

References

1. Logemann JA. Evaluation and Treatment of Swallowing Disorders. Austin, TX: Pro-Ed; 1998.

2. Sizoo EM, Braam L, Postma TJ, et al. Symptoms and problems in the end-of-life phase of high grade glioma patients. Neuro Oncol. 2010;12(11):1162–1166.

3. Spataro R, Ficano L, Piccoli F, LaBella V. Percutaneous endoscopic gastrostomy in amyotrophic lateral sclerosis: effect on survival. J Neurol Sci. 2011;304(1–2):44.

4. Hill M, Hughes T, Milford C. Treatment for swallowing difficulties (dysphagia) in chronic muscle disease. Cochrane Database Syst Rev. 2004(2):CD004303.

5. American Geriatrics Society. Feeding Tubes in Advanced Dementia Position Statement. New York, NY: American Geriatrics Society; 2013.

6. Sura L, Madhavan A, Carnaby G, Crary MA. Dysphagia in the elderly: management and nutritional considerations. Clin Interv Aging. 2012;7:287–298.

7. Altman K, Yu G, Schaefer S. Consequence of dysphagia in the hospitalized patient: impact on prognosis and hospital resources. Arch Otolaryngol Head Neck Surg. 2010;136(8):784–789.

8. Logemann JA, Gensler G, Robbins J, et al. A randomized study of three interventions for aspiration of thin liquids in patients with dementia or Parkinson's disease. JSLHR. 2008;51(1):173–183.

9. Heiss CJ, Goldberg L, Dzarnoski M. Registered dietitians and speech-language pathologists: an important partnership in dysphagia management. J Am Diet Assoc. 2010;110(9):1290–1293.

10. Geeganage C, Beavan J, Ellender S, Bath PMW. Interventions for dysphagia and nutritional support in acute and subacute stroke. Cochrane Database Syst Rev. 2012;10.

11. Ames N. Evidence to support tooth brishing in critically ill patients. Am J Crit Care. 2011;20(3):242–250.

12. Griffith R, Tengnali C. A guideline for managing medication related dysphagia. Br J Community Nurs. 2012;12(9):426–429.

13. Cai S, Gozalo P, Mitchell S, et al. Do patients with advanced cognitive impairment admitted to hospitals with higher rates of feeding tube insertion have improved survival? J Pain Symptom Manage. 2013;45(3):524–533.

14. Davies A, Hall S. Salivary gland dysfunction (dry mouth) in patients with cancer. Int J Palliat Nurs. 2011;17(10):477–482.

15. Alt-Epping B, Nejad RK, Jung K, Gross U, Nauck F. Symptoms of the oral cavity and their association with local microbiological and clinical findings: a prospective survey in palliative care. Support Care Cancer. 2012;20(3):531–537.

16. Wilberg P, Hjermstad MJ, Ottesen S, Herlofson BB. Oral health is an important issue in end-of-life cancer care. Support Care Cancer. 2012;20(12):3115–3122.

17. Berti-Couto Sde A, Couto-Souza PH, Jacobs R, et al. Clinical diagnosis of hyposalivation in hospitalized patients. J Appl Oral Sci. 2012;20(2):157–161.

18. Bryan G, Furness S, Birchenough S, McMillan R, Worthington HV. Interventions for the management of dry mouth: nonpharmacological interventions. Cochrane Database Syst Rev. 2012(2).

19. Fehrenbach M. American Dental Hygienists' Assocation Hyposalivation with Xerostomia Screening Tool: Access. 2010. http://www.adha.org/resources-docs/72614_Access_Hyposalivation_Tool.pdf. Accessed October 30, 2013.

20. Wiener RC, Wu B, Crout R, et al. Hyposalivation and xerostomia in dentate older adults. J Am Dent Assoc. 2010;141(3):279–284.

21. Cancer Care Ontario, Action Cancer Ontario. Xerostomia. Symptom management guides 2013. https://www.cancercare.on.ca/toolbox/symptools/.

22. Dahlin C, Cohen A, Goldsmith, T. Dysphagia, xerostomia, and hiccups. In: BR Ferrell, N Coyle (eds.), Oxford Textbook of Palliative Nursing. New York, NY: Oxford University Press; 2010:239–267.

23. American Cancer Society. External Radiation Side Effects Worksheet. 2013. http://www.cancer.org/acs/groups/content/@nho/documents/document/acsq-009503.pdf. Accessed June 22, 2013.

24. Oncology Nursing Society. Radiation Therapy Patient Care Record. Pittsburgh: PA: Oncology Nursing Society Press, 2002.

25. Furness S, Worthington HV, Bryan G, Birchenough S, McMillan R. Interventions for the management of dry mouth: topical therapies (Review). Cochrane Database Syst Rev. 2011;12.

26. Meng Z, Garcia K, Hu C, et al. Randomized controlled trial of acupuncture for prevention of radiation-induced xerostomia among patients with nashopharyngeal carcinoma. Cancer. 2012;118(13):3337–3344.

27. Calsina-Berna A, Garcia-Gomez G, Gonzalez-Barboteo J, Porta-Sales J. Treatment of chronic hiccups in cancer patients: a systematic review [Review]. J Palliat Med. 2012;15(10):1142–1150.

28. Moretto EN, Wee B, Wiffen PJ, Murchison AG. Interventions for treating persistent and intractable hiccups in adults. [Review]. Cochrane Database Syst Rev. 2013;1.

29. Porzio G, Aielli F, Verna L, Aloisi P, Galletti B, C F. Gabapentin in the treatment of hiccups in patients with advanced cancer: a 5-year experience. Clin Neuropharmacol. 2010;33(4):179–180.

Chapter 5

Bowel Management

Constipation, Diarrhea, Obstruction, and Ascites

Denice Caraccia Economou

Constipation

Functional constipation affects 30% of the general population.[1] The incidence may be as high as 30% to 100% in palliative care patients. Constipation is a major problem in cancer patients and is responsible for great amounts of suffering and embarrassment. The use of opioids for pain contributes to constipation, and this side effect is the principal reason for their discontinuation. Constipation is common, yet prophylactic treatment is inconsistently begun by both physicians and nurses.

Definitions

Constipation is subjective to many patients, making assessment difficult. Constipation is defined as a decrease in the frequency of passage of formed stools and is characterized by stools that are hard and small and difficult to expel.

Associated symptoms of constipation vary, but may include:

- Excessive straining
- A feeling of fullness or pressure in the rectum
- The sensation of incomplete emptying
- Abdominal distention
- Cramps

In an effort to establish a validated and objective way to define functional constipation and develop a scientific approach to understanding and treating functional gastrointestinal disorders (FGIDs) researchers developed the first Rome I in 1994. They have expanded their classification system with scientific evidence and continue to use scientific evidence to promote the best treatment for FGIDs. The Rome III criteria were established in 2007 and are used in many palliative care settings. Patients are constipated if they experience at least two of the following symptoms:

- Less than three stools per week
- Straining with at least 25% of stools
- Lumpy, hard stool at least 25% of the time

- Feeling of incomplete evacuation or sensation of blockage for at least 25% of stools
- Need to manually remove stool at least 25% of the time
- Loose stools are rarely present without the use of laxatives
- Lack of sufficient criteria for irritable bowel syndrome

The subjective experience of constipation may vary for different individuals, underscoring the importance of individualized patient assessment and management.

Prevalence and Impact

It is estimated that 54% of hospice patients are constipated; this may be an underestimate, as many of those patients are on opioids and stool softeners/laxatives at baseline. Inpatient hospitalization and ambulatory clinic visits for constipation and related side effects cost the healthcare system $235 million annually. Constipation is considered a symptom of bowel dysfunction (BD) and opioid bowel dysfunction (OBD) relating to opioid-induced constipation. The impact of constipation on quality of life is substantial. Constipation causes social, psychological, and physical distress for patients, which additionally impacts the caregiver and healthcare staff. Failure to anticipate and manage constipation in a proactive way significantly affects the difficulty a patient will experience in attempting to relieve this problem.

Pathophysiology

Normal bowel function includes three areas of control: small intestinal motility, colon motility, and defecation. This includes the processes of secretion, absorption, transport, and storage.

- Small-intestinal activity is primarily the mixing of contents by bursts of propagated motor activity that are associated with increased gastric, pancreatic, and biliary secretion. This motor activity occurs every 90 to 120 minutes, but is altered when food is ingested. Contents are mixed to allow for digestion and absorption of nutrients. When the stomach has emptied, the small intestine returns to regular propagated motor activity.

- The colon propels contents forward through peristaltic movements. The colon movement is much slower than that of the small intestine. Contents may remain in the colon for up to 2 to 3 days, whereas small-intestinal transit is 2–4 hours. Motor activity in the large intestine occurs approximately six times per day, usually grouped in two peak bursts. The first is triggered by awakening and breakfast, and a smaller burst is triggered by the afternoon meal. Contractions are stimulated by ingestion of food, psychogenic factors, and somatic activity.

- The physiology of defecation involves coordinated interaction between the involuntary internal anal sphincter and the voluntary external anal sphincter. The residual intestinal contents distend the rectum and initiate expulsion. The longitudinal muscle of the rectum contracts, and, with the voluntary external anal sphincter relaxed, defecation can occur. Additional coordinated muscle activity also occurs and includes contraction of the diaphragm against a closed glottis, tensing of the abdominal wall, and relaxation of the pelvic floor.

The enteric nervous system plays an important role in the movement of bowel contents through the gastrointestinal (GI) tract as well. Smooth muscles in the GI tract have spontaneous electrical, rhythmic activity, resembling pacemakers in the stomach and small intestine that communicate with the remainder of the bowel. There are both submucosal and myenteric plexuses of nerves. These nerves are connected to the central nervous system through sympathetic ganglia, splanchnic nerves, and parasympathetic fibers in the vagus nerve and the presacral plexus. Opioid medications affect the myenteric plexus, which coordinates peristalsis. Therefore, peristalsis is decreased and stool transit time is increased, leading to harder, dryer, and less frequent stools, or constipation. Constipation therefore is related to dysfunction of either the colon or neuromuscular system. Important factors that promote normal functioning of the bowel include the following:

1. *Fluid intake.* Nine liters of fluid (which includes 7 liters secreted from the salivary glands, stomach, pancreas, small bowel, and biliary system, and the average oral intake of 2 liters) are reduced to 1.5 liters by the time they reach the colon. At this point, water and electrolytes continue to be absorbed, and the end volume for waste is 150 mL. Decreased fluid intake may make a significant difference in the development of constipation.

2. *Adequate dietary fiber.* The presence of food in the stomach initiates the muscle contractions and secretions from the biliary, gastric, and pancreatic systems that lead to movement of the bowels. The amount of dietary fiber consumed is related to stool size and consistency. Smaller meal size also reduces the natural trigger for peristalsis, adding to constipation.

3. *Physical activity.* Colonic propulsion is related to intraluminal pressures in the colon. Lack of physical activity and reduced intraluminal pressures can significantly reduce propulsive activity. Lack of mobility may also interfere with the patient's ability to sit on the toilet because of decreased muscle mass or increased fatigue.

4. *Adequate time or privacy to defecate.* Changes in normal bowel routines, such as morning coffee or reading the paper, can decrease peristalsis and lead to constipation. Emotional disturbances are also known to affect gut motility.

Primary, Secondary, and Iatrogenic Constipation

Causes of constipation in cancer patients are divided into three different categories.

- Primary constipation is caused by reduced fluid and fiber intake, decreased activity, lack of privacy, and advanced age.
- Secondary constipation is related to structural, metabolic, or neurologic disorders. These changes may include tumor; partial intestinal obstruction; metabolic effects of hypercalcemia, hypothyroidism, hypokalemia,

or hyperglycemia; spinal cord compression at the level of the cauda equina or sacral plexus; sacral nerve infiltration; and cerebral tumors.

- Iatrogenically induced constipation is related to pharmacological interventions. Opioids are the primary medications associated with constipation.[2] In addition, chemotherapies (vincristine, oxaliplatin, temozolomide, thalidomide), anticholinergic medications (belladonna, antihistamines), antiemetic therapy (5HT-3 antagonists), tricyclic antidepressants (nortriptyline, amitriptyline), neuroleptics (haloperidol and chlorpromazine), antispasmodics, anticonvulsants (phenytoin and gabapentin), muscle relaxants, aluminum antacids, iron, diuretics (furosemide), and antiparkinsonian agents cause constipation.[3]

Constipation Related to Cancer and Its Treatment

Multiple factors associated with cancer and its treatment cause constipation.

- Cancers involving the GI system or those anatomically associated with the bowel, cause constipation.
- Pelvic cancers, including ovarian, cervical, and uterine cancers, are highly associated with constipation and mechanical obstruction.
- Malignant ascites, spinal cord compression, and paraneoplastic autonomic neuropathy also cause constipation.
- Cancer-related causes include surgical interruption of the GI tract, decreased activity, reduced intake of both fluids and food, changes in personal routines associated with bowel movements, bed rest, confusion, and depression.

Opioid-Related Constipation

Opioids affect bowel function primarily by inhibiting propulsive peristalsis through the small bowel and colon. Chronic opioid use in noncancer patients causes constipation in 40% of the patients; in advanced cancer patients, 50% to 90% will develop bowel dysfunction.

- Opioids bind with the receptors on the smooth muscles of the bowel, affecting the contraction of the circular and longitudinal muscle fibers that cause peristalsis or the movement of contents through the bowel.
- Colonic transit time is lengthened, contributing to increased fluid and electrolyte absorption and dryer, harder stools.
- Peristaltic changes occur 5 to 25 minutes after administration of the opioid and are dose related.
- Patients do not develop tolerance to the constipation side effects even with long-term use of opioids.

Assessment of Constipation

History

Managing constipation requires a thorough history and physical examination.[4] The lack of a universally accepted definition of constipation complicates diagnosis and management. Evidence has shown that healthcare providers cannot diagnose constipation in an objective way. Finding a tool to help establish a method to identify and stage constipation to aid in prophylactic management is essential.

The Constipation Assessment Scale (CAS) was developed in 1989 and has been tested for validity and reliability and found to have a significant ability to differentiate the severity of constipation between moderate and severe constipation. It uses the criteria of the ROME III to define functional constipation. It is a simple questionnaire that requires on average 2 minutes to complete (Table 5.1).[5] The CAS includes eight symptoms associated with constipation:

- Abdominal distention or bloating
- Change in amount of gas passed rectally
- Less frequent bowel movements
- Oozing liquid stool
- Rectal fullness or pressure
- Rectal pain with bowel movement
- Small volume of stool
- Inability to pass stool

These symptoms are rated as 0, not experienced; 1, some problem; or 2, severe problem. A score between 0 and 16 is calculated and can be used as an objective measurement of subjective symptoms for ongoing management.

It is important to start by asking patients when they moved their bowels last and to follow up by asking what their normal movement pattern is. Remember, what is considered constipated for one person is not for someone else.

- What are the characteristics of their stools and did they note any blood or mucus?
- Were their bowels physically difficult to move? This is especially important if they have cancer in or near the intestines or rectal area that may contribute to physical obstruction.

Table 5.1 Constipation Assessment Scale
Direction: Circle the appropriate number to indicate whether, during the past 3 days, you have had **NO PROBLEM**, **SOME PROBLEM**, or a **SEVERE PROBLEM** with each of the items listed

Item	No Problem	Some Problem	Severe Problem
1. Abdominal distention or bloating	0	1	2
2. Change in amount of gas passed rectally	0	1	2
3. Less frequent bowel movements	0	1	2
4. Oozing liquid stool	0	1	2
5. Rectal fullness or pressure	0	1	2
6. Rectal pain with bowel movement	0	1	2
7. Smaller stool size	0	1	2
8. Urge but inability to pass stool	0	1	2
Patient's Name			Date

Reproduced with permission from McMillan SC, Williams FA. Validity and reliability of the Constipation Assessment Scale. Cancer Nurs. 1989;12(3):183–188.

- Do they feel bloated or is there pressure in the abdomen?
- Does the patient feel pain when moving the bowels?
- Is the patient oozing liquid stool?
- Does the patient feel that the volume of stool passed is small?
- Are they experiencing nausea that cannot be explained?

Medication- or Disease-Related History

The patient's medical status and anticipated disease process are important in providing insight into areas where early intervention could prevent severe constipation or even obstruction. Box 5.1 lists more common causes of constipation in palliative care.

Physical Examination

Begin the physical examination in the mouth, to ensure that the patient is able to chew foods and that there are no lesions or tumors in the mouth that could interfere with eating. Does the patient wear dentures? Patients who wear dentures and have lost a great deal of weight may have dentures that do not fit properly, which would make eating and drinking difficult.

Abdominal Examination

- Inspect the abdomen initially for bloating, distention, or bulges. Distention may be associated with obesity, fluid, tumor, or gas. Remember, the patient should have emptied the bladder.
- Auscultation is important to evaluate the presence or absence of bowel sounds. If no bowel sounds are audible initially, listen continuously for a minimum of 5 minutes. The absence of bowel sounds may indicate a paralytic ileus. If the bowel sounds are hyperactive, it could indicate diarrhea. Percussion of the bowel may result in tympany, which is related to gas in the bowel. A dull sound is heard over intestinal fluid and feces.
- Palpation of the abdomen should start lightly; look for muscular resistance and abdominal tenderness. This is usually associated with chronic constipation. If rebound tenderness is detected with coughing or light palpation, peritoneal inflammation should be considered. Deep palpation may reveal a "sausage-like" mass of stool in the left colon. Feeling stool in the colon indicates constipation.
- A digital examination of the rectum may reveal stool or possible tumor or rectocele. If the patient is experiencing incontinence of liquid stool, obstruction must be considered. Examining for hemorrhoids, ulcerations, or rectal fissures is important, especially in the neutropenic patient. Patients with neutropenia can complain of rectal pain well before a rectal infection is obvious. Evaluating the patient for infection, ulceration, or rectal fissures is very important. Additionally, determine whether the patient has had previous intestinal surgery, alternating diarrhea and constipation, complaints of abdominal colic pain or nausea, and vomiting.
- Examining the stool for shape and consistency can also be useful. Stools that are hard and pelletlike suggest slow transit time, whereas stools that are ribbonlike suggest hemorrhoids. Blood or mucus in the stool suggests tumor, hemorrhoids, or possibly preexisting colitis.

Box 5.1 Causes of Constipation in Cancer/Palliative Care Patients

Etiology

Cancer Related

Directly related to tumor site. Primary bowel cancers, secondary bowel cancers, pelvic cancers.

Surgical interruption of bowel integrity.

Intestinal obstruction related to tumor in the bowel wall or external compression by tumor.

Damage to the lumbosacral spinal cord, cauda equina, or pelvic plexus.

High spinal cord transection mainly stops the motility response to food.

Low spinal cord or pelvic outflow lesions produce dilation of the colon and slow transit in the descending and distal transverse colon.

Surgery in the abdomen can lead to adhesion development or direct changes in the bowel.

Hypercalcemia

Cholinergic control of secretions of the intestinal epithelium is mediated by changes in intracellular calcium concentrations.

Hypercalcemia causes decreased absorption, leading to constipation, whereas hypercalcemia can lead to diarrhea.

Secondary Effects Related to the Disease

Decreased appetite, decreased fluid intake, low-fiber diet, weakness, inactivity, confusion, depression, change in normal toileting habits.

Decreased fluid and food intake leading to dehydration and weakness.

Decreased intake, ineffective voluntary elimination actions, as well as decreased normal defecation reflexes.

Decreased peristalsis; increased colonic transit time leads to increased absorption of fluid and electrolytes and small, hard, dry stools.

Inactivity, weakness, changes in normal toileting habits, daily bowel function reflexes, and positioning affect ability to use abdominal wall musculature and relax pelvic floor for proper elimination.

Psychological depression can increase constipation by slowing down motility.

Concurrent Disease

Diabetes (hyperglycemia), hypothyroidism, hypokalemia, diverticular disease, hemorrhoids, colitis, chronic neurological diseases.

Electrolytes and therefore water are transported via neuronal control. Like hypercalcemia, abnormal potassium can affect water absorption and contribute to constipation. Chronic neurological diseases affect the neurological stimulation of intestinal motility.

(Continued)

Box 5.1 (Continued)

Medication Related

Opioid medications

Anticholinergic effects (hydroscine, phenothiazines)

Tricyclic antidepressants

Antiparkinsonian drugs

Iron

Antihypertensives, antihistamines

Antacids

Diuretics

Vinca alkaloid chemotherapy

Management of Constipation

Preventing constipation whenever possible is the most important management strategy.[4] Constipation can be extremely distressing to many patients and severely affects quality of life. The complicating factor remains the individuality of a patient's response to constipation therapy. Therefore, there is no set rule for the most effective way to manage constipation.

Improving three important primary causes of constipation is essential.

- Encouraging fluid intake is a priority. Increasing or decreasing fluid intake by as little as 100 mL can affect constipation.

- Increase dietary intake as much as possible, although this is difficult for many patients. Focusing on food intake for some patients can increase their anxiety and discomfort. Increasing the fiber intake for patients in general may be helpful, but in palliative care, high fiber in the diet can cause more discomfort and constipation. Fiber without fluid absorbs what little liquid the patient may have available in the bowel and makes the bowels more difficult to move. For example, caution is needed for patients who use bulk laxatives such as psyllium, especially if they are not taking sufficient fluid intake.

- Encouraging activity whenever possible, even in end-of-life care, can be very helpful. Increased activity helps to stimulate peristalsis and to improve mood. Physical therapy should be used as part of a multidisciplinary bowel-management approach. Providing basic range of motion, either active or passive, can improve bowel management and patient satisfaction.

Pharmacological Management

Types of Laxatives

Laxatives can be classified by their actions.

Bulk Laxatives: Bulk laxatives provide bulk to the intestines to increase mass, stimulating the bowel to move. Increasing dietary fiber is considered a bulk laxative. The recommended dose of bran is 8 g daily. Other bulk laxatives include psyllium, carboxymethylcellulose, and methylcellulose. Psyllium is recommended at 2 to 4 teaspoons daily as a bulk laxative; action may take 2 to 3 days.

- Bulk laxatives are more helpful for mild constipation.
- It is recommended that the patient increase fluids by 200 to 300 mL when using bulk laxatives.
- The consistency of bulk laxatives is often unacceptable.
- The benefits of bulk laxatives in severe constipation are questionable.
- Additional complications include allergic reactions, fluid retention, and hyperglycemia.
- Bulk laxatives produce gas as the indigestible or nonsoluble fiber breaks down or ferments; this can cause uncomfortable bloating.

Lubricant Laxatives: Mineral oil can lubricate the stool surface and soften the stool by penetration, leading to an easier bowel movement. However, mineral oil:

- Can cause seepage from the rectum and perineal irritation
- Can lead to malabsorption of fat-soluble vitamins (vitamins A, D, E, and K)
- Can cause aspiration pneumonitis or lipoid pneumonia in the frail and elderly patient
- *For these reasons mineral oil is rarely recommended.*

Surfactant/Detergent Laxatives: Surfactant/detergent laxatives, such as docusate, reduce surface tension, which increases absorption of water and fats into dry stools, leading to a softening effect. These encourage secretion of water, sodium, and chloride in the jejunum and colon and decreases electrolyte and water reabsorption in the small and large intestines. At higher doses, these laxatives may stimulate peristalsis.

- Docusate is used alone or in combination with laxatives such as sennosides (Peri-Colace or Senokot S).
- The recommended dosage of docusate sodium is 50–500 mg daily and for docusate calcium 240 mg daily.
- Castor oil also works like a detergent laxative by exerting a surface-wetting action on the stool and directly stimulates the colon, but its use in cancer-related constipation is discouraged because results are difficult to control.

Combination Medications: Combination softener/laxative medications have been shown to be more effective than softeners alone at a lower total dose. The recommended dosage of senna/docusate is two tablets daily to twice a day.

Osmotic Laxatives: Osmotic laxatives are nonabsorbable sugars that exert an osmotic effect in both the small and, to a lesser extent, large intestines. They increase fluid secretions in the small intestines by retaining fluid in the bowel lumen. They have the additional effect of lowering ammonia levels. This is helpful in improving confusion, especially in hepatic failure patients. Laxatives in this category include: lactulose, magnesium citrate, magnesium hydroxide (milk of magnesia), polyethylene glycol (PEG 3350, MiraLax), and sodium biphosphate (Phospho-Soda). These laxatives can be effective for chronic constipation, especially when related to opioid use. Onset of action is between 2 and 48 hours.

- Drawbacks of agents like lactulose are that effectiveness is completely dose related and, for some patients, the sweet taste is intolerable. The bloating and gas associated with higher doses may be too uncomfortable or distressing to tolerate. Lactulose can be put into juice or other liquid to lessen the taste. The recommended dosage of lactulose is 30 to 60 mL initially for severe constipation every 4 hours until a bowel movement occurs. Once that happens, calculate the amount of lactulose used to achieve that movement, and then divide in half for recommended daily maintenance dose. An example: It took 60 mL to have a bowel movement; therefore, 30 mL daily should keep the bowels moving regularly.
- The recommended dosage of milk of magnesia is 30 mL to initiate a bowel movement. For opioid-related constipation, 15 mL of milk of magnesia may be added to the baseline bowel medications either daily or every other day.
- Magnesium citrate comes in a 10-ounce bottle. For severe constipation, it is used as a one-time initial therapy and is contraindicated in obstruction.
- Polyethylene glycol (PEG 3350; MiraLax, Movical [UK]) is used frequently and can be sprinkled over food. Recommended dose is 1 tablespoon/day. Evacuation can take between 2 to 4 days.
- Osmotic rectal compounds include glycerin suppositories and sorbitol enemas.

Bowel Stimulants: Bowel stimulants work directly on the colon to increase motility. These medications stimulate the myenteric plexus to induce peristalsis. They also reduce the amount of water and electrolytes in the colon. They are divided into two groups: the diphenylmethanes and the anthraquinones. The diphenylmethanes include bisacodyl and the anthraquinones are bowel stimulants that include senna and cascara. However, cascara was removed from over-the-counter medications for the treatment of constipation although it remains available as a dietary supplement.

- Bisacodyl's action is usually 6 to 12 hours when taken orally. Rectal absorption is much faster, at 15 to 60 minutes. It is recommended that bisacodyl be taken with food, milk, or antacids to avoid gastric irritation. Bisacodyl comes in 10-mg tablets or suppositories.
- Senna can be used alone or in combination with docusate. Starting dose is typically two tablets daily with a maximum of 8/day. Senna can discolor the colon with long-term use but this is rarely a concern in palliative care. Senna tea is available in most health food stores.

Rectal Medications: Although the thought of rectal medications or enemas is unpleasant for many patients, their quick onset of action can make them more acceptable when constipation is advanced and is producing more discomfort. All rectal agents should be limited when patients are neutropenic or thrombocytopenic.

- Bisacodyl comes in 10 mg suppository for adults and 5 mg as a pediatric dose. Glycerin suppositories can help lubricate the rectal vault.

- Saline enemas are used to loosen the stool and to stimulate rectal or distal colon peristalsis. Repeated use can cause hypocalcemia and hyperphosphatemia, so it is important to use enemas cautiously. Enemas should never be considered part of a standing bowel regimen. Onset of action can be within 30 minutes.
- Oil retention enemas are particularly helpful for severely constipated patients, for whom disimpaction may be necessary. They work best when used overnight, to allow softening. Overnight retention is effective only if the patient is able to retain it that long. The general rule is that the longer the enema is retained, the better the results.
- Combining an enema with an oral saline-type cathartic (lactulose, Cephulac) is helpful when a large amount of stool is present. This may help to push the stool through the GI tract.
- If disimpaction is necessary, remember that it can be extremely painful; therefore, premedicate the patient with an opioid and consider use of a benzodiazepine to reduce anxiety.

There are few studies outlining the efficacy of one enema over another. The reported success rates for rectal enemas within 1 hour includes phosphate enemas (100%), bisacodyl suppositories (66%), and glycerine suppositories (38%). If none of the above enemas is effective, Sykes recommends rectal lavage with approximately 8 liters of warmed normal saline. It is important to remember that if a patient's constipation requires this invasive intervention, you must change the usual bowel regimen once this bowel crisis is resolved.

Recent Approaches to Constipation Management

Peripherally acting opioid antagonists have become an effective method to manage opioid-related constipation in the palliative care setting.[6]

- Oral naloxone, an opioid antagonist, has less than 1% availability systemically when given orally, due to the first-pass effect in the liver. The lack of a commercially available oral formulation means that patients must drink the solution used for parenteral administration. Doses higher than 8-12 mg have been associated with reversal of analgesia.
- Methylnaltrexone (Relistor) is an opioid antagonist that is administered subcutaneously and is indicated for the treatment of opioid-induced constipation in patients with advanced illness who are not responding to standard laxative/stimulant regimens. Results occurred on the average between 30 minutes and 4 hours. Unlike oral naloxone, it crosses the blood-brain barrier less readily so therefore is less likely to reverse centrally mediated analgesia. The cost of this class of medication is a concern, although it is cheaper than a hospital admission.

Currently new areas of research are examining the use of inadvertent medications whose side effects involve relief of constipation.

- Oral erythromycin has been shown to cause diarrhea in 50% of patients who use it as an antibiotic. Currently, researchers are investigating its use to promote diarrhea.

- Amidotrizoane (gastrografin) is an oral contrast medium that is hyper-osmolar and is used as a second-line treatment for patients who are unresponsive to common laxatives in Italy. This intervention leads to a bowel movement in about 45% of the advanced cancer patients who did not respond to their anticonstipation regimen. The benefit of this medication is that it is an oral medication and fairly inexpensive. Hydration is important for patients receiving this treatment. More research is needed.

Summary

Constipation is a major problem for palliative care patients, and is responsible for great amounts of suffering and embarrassment. Nurses have an important role in preventing and managing this symptom through thorough assessment and skilled management.

Diarrhea

Diarrhea has been a major symptom and significant problem in palliative care. Treating diarrhea requires a thorough assessment and therapy directed at the specific cause. Diarrhea is usually acute and short-lived, lasting only a few days, as opposed to chronic diarrhea, which lasts 3 weeks or more. Uncontrolled diarrhea leads to dehydration, fluid and electrolyte imbalance, and malnutrition. Like constipation, this symptom can be debilitating and can severely affect quality of life. Diarrhea can prevent patients from leaving their homes, increase weakness and dehydration, and contribute to feelings of lack of control and depression. Nurses play a significant role in educating patients and recognizing and managing diarrhea and its manifestations.

Definitions

Diarrhea is described as an increase in stool volume and liquidity resulting in three or more bowel movements per day. Secondary effects related to diarrhea include:

- Abdominal cramps
- Anxiety
- Lethargy
- Weakness
- Dehydration
- Dizziness
- Loss of electrolytes
- Skin breakdown
- Pain
- Dry mouth
- Weight loss

Acute diarrhea occurs within 24 to 48 hours of exposure to the cause and resolves in 7 to 14 days. Chronic diarrhea usually has a late onset and lasts 2 to 3 weeks, with an unidentified cause.

Prevalence and Impact

Cancer patients may have multiple causes of diarrhea. It may be due to infections or related to tumor type or its treatment. Common causes of diarrhea are chemotherapy, overuse of laxative therapy or dietary fiber. Additional causes include malabsorption disorders, motility disturbances, stress, partial bowel obstruction, enterocolic fistula, villous adenoma, endocrine-induced hypersecretion of serotonin, gastrin calcitonin, and vasoactive intestinal protein prostaglandins.

Chemotherapy-induced diarrhea may be related to one drug or compounded when two diarrheal instigating medications are given together, for example, fluorouracil and irinotecan. Irinotecan may cause delayed diarrhea starting 6–14 days after treatment. Other fluorouracil family drugs like capecitabine or taxane drugs like docetaxel will cause diarrhea as well. Newer targeted therapy drugs that can cause serious diarrhea include erlotinib and gefitinib, sorafenib, sunitinib, imatinib, and bortezomib. Excessive diarrhea can lead to dose interruption.

Diarrhea associated with radiation can occur by the second or third week of treatment and can continue after radiation has been discontinued. Radiation-induced diarrhea is related to focus of radiation and total of radiation dose. Pelvic radiation alone has been shown to cause diarrhea of any grade in up to 70% of the patients receiving it. A grade 3 or 4 diarrhea is associated with approximately 20% of those patients. Acute enteritis or proctitis can occur within the first 6 weeks of therapy and resolve between 2 and 6 months post treatment. Patients who were treated with greater than 45 Grays (GY) may develop a chronic radiation enteritis. Physical changes secondary to the radiation may cause effects for months to years after treatment.

Surgical patients who have had bowel-shortening procedures or gastrectomy related to cancer experience a "dumping syndrome," which causes severe diarrhea. This type of diarrhea is related to both osmotic and hypermotile mechanisms. Patients may experience weakness, epigastric distention, and diarrhea shortly after eating. The shortened bowel can result in a decreased absorption capacity and an imbalance in absorptive and secretory function of the intestine.

Pathophysiology

Diarrhea can be grouped into four types, each with a different mechanism: osmotic diarrhea, secretory diarrhea, hypermotile diarrhea, and exudative diarrhea. Cancer patients rarely exhibit only one type. Understanding the mechanism of diarrhea permits more rational treatment strategies.

Osmotic Diarrhea

Osmotic diarrhea is produced by intake of hyperosmolar preparations or nonabsorbable solutions such as enteral feeding solutions. Enterocolic fistula can lead to both osmotic diarrhea from undigested food entering the colon and hypermotile diarrhea. Hemorrhage into the intestine can cause an osmotic-type diarrhea because intraluminal blood acts as an osmotic laxative. Osmotic diarrhea may result from insufficient lactase when dairy products are consumed.

Secretory Diarrhea

Secretory diarrhea is most associated with chemotherapy and radiation therapy. The cause is related to mechanical damage to the epithelial crypt cells in the GI tract. The necrosis that results, along with the inflammation and ulceration of the intestinal mucosa, leads to further damage related to exposure to bile and susceptibility to opportunistic infections, atrophy of the mucosal lining, and fibrosis. This all contributes to loss of absorption due to damaged villi, causing an increase in water, electrolytes, mucus, blood, and serum to be pulled into the intestine from immature crypt cells, and increased fluid secretion, resulting in diarrhea.

Secretory diarrhea is the most difficult to control. Malignant epithelial tumors producing hormones that can cause diarrhea include metastatic carcinoid tumors, gastrinoma, and medullary thyroid cancer. The primary effect of secretory diarrhea is related to the hypersecretion stimulated by endogenous mediators that affect the intestinal transport of water and electrolytes. This results in accumulation of intestinal fluids. Diarrhea associated with graft versus host disease (GVHD) after stem cell transplantation results from mucosal damage and can produce up to 6 to 8 liters of diarrhea in 24 hours. Surgical shortening of the bowel, which reduces intestinal mucosal contact and shortens colon transit time, causing decreased reabsorption, leads to diarrhea. Active treatment requires vigorous fluid and electrolyte repletion, antidiarrheal therapy, and specific anticancer therapy.

Hypermotile Diarrhea

Partial bowel obstruction from abdominal malignancies can cause a reflex hypermotility. Enterocolic fistula can lead to diarrhea from irritative hypermotility and osmotic influence of undigested food entering the colon. Biliary or pancreatic obstruction can cause incomplete digestion of fat in the small intestine, resulting in interference with fat and bile salt malabsorption, leading to hypermotile diarrhea, also called steatorrhea. Malabsorption is related to pancreatic cancer, gastrectomy, ileal resection or colectomy, rectal cancer, pancreatic islet cell tumors, or carcinoid tumors. Chemotherapy-induced diarrhea is frequently seen with 5-fluorouracil or N-phosphonoacetyl-L-aspartate. High-dose cisplatin and irinotecan (Camptosar) cause severe hypermotility. Other chemotherapy drugs that cause diarrhea include cytosine arabinoside, nitrosourea, methotrexate, cyclophosphamide, doxorubicin, daunorubicin, hydroxyurea and biotherapy-2, interferon and topoisomerase inhibitors (capecitabine [5-FU prodrug]), and oxaliplatin.

Exudative Diarrhea

Radiation therapy of the abdomen, pelvis, or lower thoracic or lumbar spine can cause acute exudative diarrhea. The inflammation caused by radiation leads to the release of prostaglandins. Treatment using aspirin or ibuprofen was shown to reduce prostaglandin release and decrease diarrhea associated with radiation therapy.

There are multiple causes of diarrhea in palliative medicine. Concurrent diseases such as diabetes mellitus, hyperthyroidism, inflammatory bowel disease, irritable bowel syndrome, and GI infection (*Clostridium difficile*) can contribute to the development of diarrhea. Finally, the dietary influences of fruit, bran, hot spices, and alcohol, as well as over-the-counter medications, laxatives, and herbal supplements, need to be considered as sources of diarrhea.

Assessment of Diarrhea

Diarrhea assessment requires a careful history to detail the frequency and nature of the stools. The National Cancer Institute Common Terminology Criteria for Adverse Events uses a grading system from 1 to 5 (Table 5.2). This scale permits an objective score to define the severity of diarrhea.

The initial goal of assessment is to identify and treat any reversible causes of diarrhea.

- Timing: If diarrhea occurs once or twice a day, it is probably related to anal incontinence.

- Amount: Large amounts of watery stools are characteristic of colonic diarrhea.

- Character: Pale, fatty, malodorous stools, called steatorrhea, are indicative of malabsorption secondary to pancreatic or small-intestinal causes.

- Onset: If a patient who has been constipated complains of sudden diarrhea with little warning, fecal impaction with overflow is the probable cause.

Table 5.2 National Cancer Institute Common Terminology Criteria for Adverse Events Version 4.03

	National Cancer Institute Grade				
	1	2	3	4	5
Diarrhea Definition: A disorder characterized by frequent and watery bowel movements.	Increase of <4 stools per day over baseline; mild increase in ostomy output compared with baseline	Increase of 4–6 stools per day over baseline; moderate increase in ostomy output compared with baseline	Increase of >=7 stools per day over baseline; in continence; hospitalization indicated; severe increase in ostomy output compared with baseline; limiting self-care ADL	Life-threatening consequences; urgent intervention indicated	Death

- Associated symptoms: If the stools are associated with cramping and urgency, it may be the result of peristalsis-stimulating laxatives.
- Medications: Evaluate medications that the patient may be taking now or in the recent past. Is the patient on laxatives? If stools are associated with fecal leakage, it may be the result of overuse of stool-softening agents such as Colace.
- Stool cultures: Depending on the aggressiveness of the treatment plan, additional assessment could include stool smears for pus, blood, fat, ova, or parasites. Stool samples for culture and sensitivity testing may be necessary to rule out additional sources of diarrhea *C. difficile* toxin, *Giardia lamblia*, or other types of GI infection.

Multifactorial causes for diarrhea make management a challenge. Assessment is essential to rule out any causes that may be easily managed.

Management of Diarrhea

The goal of diarrhea management should focus on minimizing or eliminating the factors causing the diarrhea, providing dietary interventions, and maintaining fluid and electrolyte balance as appropriate. Quality-of-life issues include minimizing skin breakdown or infections, relieving pain associated with frequent diarrhea, and maintaining the patient's dignity. A combination of supportive care and medication may be appropriate for palliative management of diarrhea.

Fluids and Food

If the patient is dehydrated, oral fluids are recommended over the IV route. Oral fluids should contain electrolytes and a source of glucose to facilitate active electrolyte transport (Box 5.2). Foods to be avoided in patients experiencing acute diarrhea include:

- Spicy food
- High-fat and fried foods
- Gas-causing foods
- Alcohol
- Caffeine
- High-sorbitol fruit and juices
- Milk and dairy products (for some patients)

Following resolution of diarrhea, the diet should start with clear liquids, flat lemonade, ginger ale, and toast or simple carbohydrates. It is recommended that the patient avoid milk if diarrhea is related to infection due to

Box 5.2 Homemade Electrolyte Replacement Solution for Adults[7]	
Adult Homemade Electrolyte Replacement Solution	
1 tsp salt	6 oz. frozen orange juice concentrate
1 tsp baking soda	6 cups water
1 tsp corn syrup	47 kcal/cup, 515 mg Na^+, 164 mg K^+

acute lactase deficiency. Protein and fats can be added to the diet slowly as diarrhea resolves.

Medication Recommendations

There are many nonspecific diarrhea medications that should be used unless infections are suspected as the cause. If *Shigella* or *C. difficile* are responsible, nonspecific antidiarrheal medications can make the diarrhea worse.

- Loperamide (Imodium) has become the drug of choice for the treatment of nonspecific diarrhea. It is a long-acting opioid agonist. The 2-mg dose has the same antidiarrheal action as 5 mg of diphenoxylate, or 45 mg of codeine. The usual management of diarrhea begins with 4 mg of loperamide, with one capsule following each loose bowel movement. Most diarrhea is managed by loperamide 2 to 4 mg once to twice a day.

- Diphenoxylate (Lomotil 2.5 mg with atropine 0.025 mg) is given as one or two tablets orally as needed for loose stools, maximum of eight/day. Diphenoxylate is derived from meperidine and binds to opioid receptors to reduce diarrhea. Atropine was added to this antidiarrheal to prevent abuse.[3] Diphenoxylate is not recommended for patients with advanced liver disease because it may precipitate hepatic coma in patients with cirrhosis. Neither diphenoxylate nor loperamide is recommended for use in children under 12 years old.

- Codeine or other opioids can be helpful.

- Tincture of opium works to decrease peristalsis, given at 0.6 mL every 4 to 6 hours. This is a controlled substance but may also provide some pain relief.

- Absorbent agents such as pectin and methylcellulose may help provide bulk to increase consistency of the stools.

- Anticholinergic drugs such as atropine and scopolamine are useful to reduce gastric secretions and decrease peristalsis. Side effects of that class of drug can complicate their use; they include dry mouth, blurred vision, and urinary hesitancy.

- Somatostatin analogs such as octreotide (Sandostatin) are also effective for secretory diarrhea that may result from endocrine tumors, AIDS, GVHD, or post-GI resection. Octreotide is administered subcutaneously at a dose of 50 to 200 mcg two or three times per day.

- Mucosal antiprostaglandin agents such as aspirin, indomethacin, and bismuth subsalicylate (Pepto-Bismol) are useful for diarrhea related to enterotoxic bacteria, radiotherapy, and prostaglandin-secreting tumors.

- Ranitidine is a useful adjuvant to octreotide for patients with Zollinger-Ellison syndrome with gastrin-induced gastric hypersecretion. Side effects include nausea and pain at injection site. Patients may also experience abdominal or headache pain.

- Clonidine is effective at controlling watery diarrhea in patients with bronchogenic cancer. Clonidine effects an alpha-2 adrenergic stimulation of electrolyte absorption in the small intestine.

- Streptozocin is used for watery diarrhea from pancreatic islet cell cancer because it decreases intestinal secretions.
- Pancreatin is a combination of amylase, lipase, and protease that is available for pancreatic enzyme replacement. It is generally administered before meals.
- Lactaid may also be helpful for malabsorption-related diarrhea.
- See Box 5.3 for medications and foods to avoid in the treatment of cancer-related diarrhea.

Nursing Interventions for Diarrhea

Nursing interventions should include nonpharmacological interventions focused on diet and psychosocial support (Box 5.4).

Summary

Managing diarrhea in the palliative care patient is challenging at best. Palliative goals of diarrhea therapy should be to restore an optimal pattern of elimination, maintain fluid and electrolyte balance as desired, preserve nutritional status, protect skin integrity, and ensure the patient's comfort and dignity.

Malignant Obstruction

As primary tumors grow in the large intestine, they can lead to obstruction.[8] Obstruction is related to the site and stage of disease. Tumors in the splenic flexure obstruct 49% of the time, but those in the rectum or rectosigmoid junction only 6% of the time. Obstruction can occur intraluminally related to primary tumors of the colon. Intramural obstruction is related to tumor in the muscular layers of the bowel wall. The bowel appears thickened, indurated, and contracted. Extramural obstruction is

---

Box 5.3 Management of Cancer-Related Diarrhea: Medications and Foods to Avoid[8]

Medications to Avoid

Antibiotics, bulk laxatives (Metamucil, methylcellulose), magnesium-containing medications (Maalox, Mylanta), promotility agents (propulsid, metoclopramide), stool softeners/laxatives, herbal supplements (milk thistle, aloe, cayenne, saw palmetto, Siberian ginseng).

Foods to Avoid

Milk and dairy products (cheese, yogurt, ice cream), caffeine-containing products (coffee, tea, cola drinks, chocolate), carbonated and high-sugar or high-sorbitol juices (prune pear, sweet cherry, peach, apple, orange juice), high-fiber/gas-causing legumes (raw vegetables, whole grain products, dried legumes, popcorn), high-fat foods (fried foods, high-fat spreads, or dressings), heavily spiced foods that taste "hot."

High risk foods—sushi, street vendors, buffets.

Box 5.4 Nursing Role in the Management of Diarrhea

Environmental Assessment

- Assess the patient's and/or caregiver's ability to manage the level of care necessary.
- Evaluate home for medical equipment that may be helpful (bedpan or commode chair).

History

- Frequency of bowel movements in last 2 weeks
- Fluid intake (normal 2 quarts/day)
- Fiber intake (normal 30–40 g/day)
- Appetite and whether patient is nauseated or vomiting. Does diet include spicy foods?
- Assess for current medications the patient has taken that are associated with causing diarrhea (laxative use, chemotherapy, antibiotics, enteral nutritional supplements, nonsteroidal antiinflammatory drugs).
- Surgical history that may contribute to diarrhea (gastrectomy, pancreatectomy, bypass, or ileal resection)
- Recent radiotherapy to abdomen, pelvis, lower spine
- Cancer diagnosis associated with diarrhea includes abdominal malignancies, partial bowel obstruction; enterocolic fistulas; metastatic carcinoid tumors; gastrinomas; medullary thyroid cancer.
- Immunosuppressed, susceptible to bacterial, protozoan, and viral diseases associated with diarrhea
- Concurrent diseases associated with diarrhea: gastroenteritis, inflammatory bowel disease, irritable bowel syndrome, diabetes mellitus, lactose deficiency, hyperthyroidism

Physical Assessment

- Examine perineum or ostomy site for skin breakdown, fissures, or external hemorrhoids.
- Gentle digital rectal examination for impaction
- Abdominal examination for distention of palpable stool in large bowel
- Examine stools for signs of bleeding.
- Evaluate for signs of dehydration.

Interventions

- Treatment should be related to cause (i.e., if obstruction is cause of diarrhea, giving antidiarrheal medications would be inappropriate).
- Assist with correcting any obvious factors related to assessment (e.g., decreasing nutritional supplements, changing fiber intake, holding or substituting medications associated with diarrhea).
- If bacterial causes are suspected, notify physician and culture stools as instructed. *Clostridium difficile* is most common.

(continued)

Box 5.4 (Continued)

- Educate patient and family on importance of cleansing the perineum gently after each stool, to prevent skin breakdown. If patient has a colostomy, stomal area must also be watched closely and surrounding skin protected. Use skin barrier to protect the skin. Frequent sitz baths may be helpful.
- Instruct patient and family on signs and symptoms that should be reported to the nurse or physician: excessive thirst, dizziness, fever, palpitations, rectal spasms, excessive cramping, watery or bloody stools.

Dietary Measures

- Eat small, frequent, bland meals.
- Low-residue diet—potassium-rich (bananas, rice, peeled apples, dry toast).
- Avoid intake of hyperosmotic supplements (e.g., Ensure, Sustacal).
- Increase fluids in diet. Approximately 3 liters of fluid a day if possible. Drinking electrolyte fluids such as Pedialyte may be helpful.
- Homeopathic treatments for diarrhea include ginger tea, glutamine, and peeled apples.

Pharmacological Management

- Opioids—codeine, paregoric, diphenoxylate, loperamide, tincture of opium
- Absorbents—pectin, aluminum hydroxide
- Adsorbents—charcoal, kaolin
- Antisecretory—aspirin, bismuth subsalicylate, prednisone, Sandostatin, ranitidine hydrochloride, indomethacin
- Anticholinergics—scopolamine, atropine sulfate, belladonna
- Alpha-2-adrenergic agonists—clonidine

  Report to nurse or physician if antidiarrheal medication seems ineffective.

Psychosocial Interventions

Provide support to patient and family. Recognize negative effects of diarrhea on quality of life:
- Fatigue
- Malnutrition
- Alteration in skin integrity
- Pain and discomfort
- Sleep disturbances
- Limited ability to travel
- Compromised role within the family
- Decreased sexual activity
- Caregiver burden

related to mesenteric and omental masses and malignant adhesions. The common metastatic pattern, in relation to primary disease in the pancreas, ovaries, or stomach, generally goes to the duodenum, from the colon to the jejunum and ileum, and from the prostate or bladder to the rectum. Bowel obstruction is not always due to tumors. Hernias, radiation-induced strictures, or adhesions may be the cause, so it is important that patients with obstructive symptoms be thoroughly evaluated to rule out a correctable cause.

Definition

There is no standard definition for malignant bowel obstruction (MBO). A current definition uses the criteria that there is clinical evidence of bowel obstruction, obstruction beyond the ligament of Treitz (in the setting of intra-abdominal cancer with incurable disease), or non-intra-abdominal primary cancer with clear intraperitoneal disease. The significance of an agreed on definition is the ability to evaluate treatment plans for evidence-based recommendations.[8]

• Clinical evidence of intestinal obstruction is occlusion of the lumen or absence of the normal propulsion that affects elimination from the GI tract.

• Motility disruption, either impaired or absent, leads to a functional obstruction but without occlusion of the intestinal lumen.

• Mechanical obstruction results in the accumulation of fluids and gas proximal to the obstruction. Distention occurs as a result of intestinal gas, ingested fluids, and digestive secretions. It becomes a self-perpetuating phenomenon, as when distention increases, intestinal secretion of water and electrolytes increases. A small-bowel obstruction causes large amounts of diarrhea. The increased fluid in the bowel leads to increased peristalsis, with large quantities of bacteria growing in the intestinal fluid of the small bowel.

• Additional factors include multiple sites of obstruction along the intestine and constipating medications, fecal impaction, fibrosis, or change in normal flora of the bowel.

The goal of treatment is to prevent obstruction from happening whenever possible.

Prevalence and Impact

The best treatment options for bowel obstruction in a patient with advanced cancer remain undetermined.[9,10] Managing MBO is dependent on the level of obstruction, disease status related to prognosis, prior treatments, and the patient's current health status. As obstruction increases, bacteria levels increase and can lead to sepsis and associated multisystem failure and death.[9]

Bowel obstruction can occur in between 5% and 43% of patients with advanced disease. Intestinal obstruction related to benign causes in patients with a previous malignancy can be significant: 3%–48%. Patients with a history of cancer who present with symptoms of bowel obstruction should be evaluated both clinically and radiologically. Each case must be evaluated individually with care decisions based on goal of treatment. Unfortunately, studies also differ in defining a successful outcome. Defining success may be evaluated based on:

- Ability to resume oral intake
- Relief of pain, nausea, or vomiting
- Extended survival
- Improvement in quality of life

Assessment and Management of Malignant Obstruction

Patients may experience severe nausea, vomiting, and abdominal pain associated with a partial or complete bowel obstruction. In the elderly patient, fecal impaction may also cause urinary incontinence. General signs and symptoms associated with different sites of obstruction are listed in Table 5.3.[9]

Providing thoughtful and supportive interventions may be more appropriate than aggressive, invasive procedures. The signs and symptoms of obstruction may be acute, with nausea, vomiting, and abdominal pain. A majority of the time, however, obstruction is a slow and insidious phenomenon, which may progress from partial to complete obstruction. Palliative care should allow for a thoughtful and realistic approach to management of obstruction within the goals of care. Treatment options start with a nonsurgical approach, and emergent surgical intervention is usually not necessary unless the risk of perforation is imminent.

Radiological Examination

Radiological examination should be limited unless surgery is being considered. Bowel obstruction may be diagnosed on the basis of a plain abdominal X-ray, but contrast may help identify the site and extent of the obstruction. Exams using CT have shown an accuracy of 94% in determining the cause of a bowel obstruction. The use of either CT or MRI to help develop a treatment plan for MBO has improved decision-making between a surgical or medical management approach. Barium is not recommended because it may interfere with additional studies.

Table 5.3 Sites of Intestinal Obstruction and Related Side Effects	
Site	**Side Effects**
Duodenum	Severe vomiting with large amounts of undigested food. Bowel sounds: succussion splash may be present. No pain or distention noted. Anorexia present
Small intestine	Moderate to severe vomiting; usually hyperactive bowel sounds with borborygmi; pain in upper and central abdomen, colic in nature; moderate distention. Periumbilical pain
Large intestine	Vomiting is a late side effect. Borborygmi bowel sounds, severe distention. Pain central to lower abdomen, colic in nature.

Ripamonti CI. Malignant bowel obstruction: tailoring treatment to individual patients. J Support Oncol. 2008;6(3):114–115.

Surgical Intervention

When considering a surgical intervention, a thorough assessment of prognostic factors is needed. These factors include:

- General medical condition
- Advanced age
- Performance status
- Psychological health
- Social support
- Tumor grade
- Poor nutritional status
- Ascites
- Palpable abdominal masses
- Distant metastases
- Previous radiation to the abdomen or pelvis
- Combination chemotherapy
- Multiple small-bowel obstructions

Other questions include:

- Will the procedure relieve symptoms for an extended amount of time with reasonable operative morbidity?
- What are the risks and benefits of the surgery in contrast to nonsurgical options?
- What are the patient's goals?

Improved options for management of MBO have developed as pharmacology and interventional radiology have been included in palliative care options. Advancements in imaging have improved the diagnosis of the cause of the MBO to help choose more appropriate interventions. This is especially important in light of the high morbidity and mortality associated with surgery in this population.

Alternative Interventions

Less invasive techniques when compared with major surgery include nasogastric or nasointestinal tubes, which can be used to decompress the bowel and/or stomach.[11] Use of these interventions, although uncomfortable for the patient, has been suggested for symptom relief while evaluating the possibility of surgery. Venting gastrostomy or jejunostomy can be a relatively easy alternative, which is especially effective for severe nausea and vomiting. It can be placed percutaneously with sedation and local anesthesia. Patients can then be fed a liquid diet, with the tube clamped for as long as tolerated without nausea or vomiting.[8]

Endoscopic Palliation

Laparoscopic surgical techniques have brought about new options for inoperable cancers. Gastroenterologists or interventional radiologists now have an increased role in palliating obstructions. The use of enteral self-expandable metal stents (SEMS) is a permanent intervention performed through endoscopy to improve luminal patency and allow oral intake without surgery. The use of SEMS has been highly effective for MBO and, in some cases, has prevented the need for colostomy. Placement is usually done in interventional radiology and requires close clinical observation, since perforation is a potential complication. It allows emergent relief of obstruction and may be the best option for palliative care patients with poor prognosis.

Complications of stent placement are divided into early or late effects. Early is related to stent misdeployment or malpositioning or perforation. Late complications include tumor growth extending through the stent into the lumen, stent migration, bleeding, or perforation.

Decompression Tubes

Colonic decompression tubes are used to reduce acutely distended bowel to prevent perforation and prevent more invasive surgical procedures. They can be placed by endoscopy or over a guidewire. They are inexpensive and widely available and prevent surgical intervention with colostomy. Disadvantages include success being dependent on the person placing them and the risk of dislodgment of the tubes. The size of these tubes allows for bowel cleansing or stool removal. These tubes are recommended as a temporizing measure to relieve distention and hopefully allow for bowel cleaning. More research needs to be done on the success of these larger decompression tubes.

Symptom Therapy

Providing aggressive pharmacological management of the distressing symptoms associated with MBO can prevent the need for surgical intervention. The symptoms of intestinal colic, vomiting, and diarrhea can be effectively controlled with medications for most patients. The goal of pharmacological symptom management in inoperable patients should be aimed at:

- Relieving abdominal pain and intestinal colic
- Reducing nausea and vomiting
- Preventing the need for a nasogastric tube
- Allowing the patient to return home, optimally with hospice care

Depending on the location of the obstruction, either high or low, symptom severity can be affected. As accumulation of secretions increases, abdominal pain also increases. Distention, vomiting, and prolonged constipation occur. With high obstruction, onset of vomiting is sooner and amounts are larger. Intermittent borborygmi and visible peristalsis may occur. Patients may experience colic pain on top of continuous pain from a growing mass. In chronic bowel obstruction, colic pain subsides. There are multiple options to attempt in an effort to relieve the symptoms and obstruction of an MBO (Box 5.5).

Antisecretory Drugs

Octreotide may be an option in early management to prevent partial obstructions from becoming complete.[10] Although octreotide is used for diarrhea because it decreases peristalsis, it also slows the irregular and ineffective peristaltic movements of obstruction, reducing the activity and balancing out the intestinal movement. It reduces vomiting because

Box 5.5 Obstruction Management Options[9,10]

1. Prevent obstruction if at all possible
2. Octreotide—0.2–0.9 mg/day IV or SQ. May prevent complete obstruction if used early
3. Opioids IV/SQ relieve pain
4. Antiemetic medications—haloperidol 5–15 mg/day, metoclopromide 10 mg Q 4 h. SQ—only if no colicky pain. Prochlorperazine 25–75 mg/day rectally, chlorpromazine 50–100 mg rectally/subcutaneous Q 8 h
5. Anticholinergics—scopolamine butybromide 40–120 mg/day, scopolamine hydrobromide 0.8–2.0 mg/day
6. Corticosteroids
7. Fluids and nutrients as tolerated
8. Laxative medications—stimulating laxatives **contraindicated** due to ↑ peristalsis. Stool softener meds may be helpful if a partial obstruction only.
9. Antidiarrheal medications—subacute obstruction or fecal fistula—codeine, loperamide, or octreotide
10. Endoscopic therapeutic devices—self-expandable metal stents (SEMS)
11. Colonic decompression tubes
12. Surgery

it inhibits the secretion of gastrin, secretin, vasoactive intestinal peptide, pancreatic polypeptide, insulin, and glucagon. Octreotide directly blocks the secretion of gastric acid, pepsin, pancreatic enzyme, bicarbonate, intestinal epithelial electrolytes, and water. It has been shown to be effective in 60% of patients for the control of vomiting. Octreotide is administered by SQ infusion or SQ injection every 12 hours. A negative aspect of this drug is its cost. It is expensive and requires SQ injections or SQ or IV infusions over days to weeks. The recommended starting dose is 0.3 mg/day and may increase to 0.6 mg/day. Hyoscine butylbromide is thought to be as effective as octreotide at reducing GI secretions and motility. Hyoscine butylbromide is less sedating, since it is thought to cross the blood-brain barrier less due to its low lipid solubility (see "Antispasmodic Medications").

Analgesic Medications

Opioid medications have been used to relieve pain associated with obstruction. Providing the opioid through SQ or IV infusion via a patient-controlled analgesic (PCA) pump is beneficial for two reasons: Patients may receive improved pain relief over the oral route due to improved absorption and, given access to a PCA pump, patients are allowed some control over their pain management. Alternative routes of opioid administration, such as rectal or transdermal, may also be effective.

Antiemetic Medications

The addition of the selective serotonin antagonists, the 5-hydroxytryptamine blockers (5HT-3), has made a significant difference in the treatment of nausea, especially when combined with corticosteroids for chemotherapy-induced nausea. Metoclopramide at 10 mg Q 4 hours SQ, has been the drug of choice for patients with incomplete bowel obstruction without colicky pain. It stimulates the stomach to empty its contents into the reservoir of the bowel. Once complete obstruction is present, metoclopramide is discontinued and haloperidol or another antiemetic medication is started. Haloperidol is less sedating than other antiemetic or antihistamine medications. The usual dose ranges from 5 to 15 mg/day, and at some institutions it is combined with cyclizine. Corticosteroids are particularly helpful antiemetics, especially when related to chemotherapy.

Corticosteroid Medications

Corticosteroids have been helpful as antiemetic medications. The recommended dose of dexamethasone is between 6 and 16 mg/day; the prednisolone dose starts at 50 mg/day (injection or SQ infusion). Steroids increase absorption of water and salt and reduce water and electrolytes in the intestine.

Antispasmodic Medications

Colic pain results from increased peristalsis against the resistance of a mechanical obstruction. Analgesics alone may not be effective. Hyoscine butylbromide has been used to relieve spasmlike pain and to reduce emesis. Dosing starts at 60 mg/day and increases up to 380 mg/day given by SQ infusion. Side effects are related to the anticholinergic effects, including tachycardia, dry mouth, sedation, and hypotension. Using methods to relieve dry mouth with sips of oral fluids, ice chips, and good mouth care is important.

Laxative Medications

Stimulant laxatives are contraindicated due to increased peristalsis against an obstruction. Stool-softening medications may be helpful if there is only a partial obstruction in the colon or rectum.

Summary

Helping families cope with symptoms associated with obstruction is important. Historically, the management of obstruction involved aggressive surgical intervention or symptom management alone. The initial assessment should include: (1) evaluating constipation, (2) evaluating for surgery, (3) providing pain management, and (4) managing nausea with metoclopramide. If incomplete obstruction, use dexamethasone, haloperidol, dimenhydrinate, chlorpromazine, or hyoscine butylbromide. The introduction of medications, such as octreotide, as well as newer antiemetics, has made a difference in the quality of life a patient with an MBO may experience. The important thing to remember is that the treatment plan must always be in agreement with the patient's wishes and promotion of quality of life. Discussing the patient's understanding of the situation and the options available are essential to effective and thoughtful care of bowel obstruction in the palliative care patient.

Ascites

Ascites associated with malignancy results from a combination of impaired fluid efflux and increased fluid influx. The effect of the accumulation of fluids leads to symptoms of abdominal distention, pain, nausea, early satiety, dyspnea, and reduced mobility.[12] Extreme ascites can lead to vomiting caused by external pressure on the stomach or intestines.

Ascites may be divided into three different types:

- *Central ascites* is the result of tumor-invading hepatic parenchyma, resulting in compression of the portal venous and/or the lymphatic system. There is a decrease in oncotic pressure as a result of limited protein intake and the catabolic state associated with cancer.

- *Peripheral ascites* is related to deposits of tumor cells found on the surface of the parietal or visceral peritoneum. The result is a mechanical interference with venous and/or lymphatic drainage. There is blockage at the level of the peritoneal space rather than the liver parenchyma. Macrophages increase capillary permeability and contribute to greater ascites.

- *Mixed type ascites* is a combination of central and peripheral ascites. Therefore, both compression of the portal venous and lymphatic systems and tumor cells in the peritoneum are involved. Chylous malignant ascites occurs when tumor infiltration of the retroperitoneal space causes obstruction of lymph flow through the lymph nodes and/or the pancreas.[12]

Additional sources of ascites not related to malignancy include the following:

- Preexisting advanced liver disease with portal hypertension
- Portal venous thrombosis
- Congestive heart failure
- Nephrotic syndrome
- Pancreatitis
- Tuberculosis
- Hepatic venous obstruction
- Bowel perforation

Severe ascites is associated with poor prognosis (40% 1-year survival, less than 10% 3-year survival). The pathological mechanisms of malignant ascites make the prevention or reduction of abdominal fluid accumulation difficult. Invasive management of ascites is seen as appropriate based on extent of ascites, prognosis, and etiology of disease. Although survival is limited, the effects of ascites on the patient's quality of life warrant an aggressive approach.

Tumor types most associated with ascites include:

- Ovarian
- Endometrial

- Breast
- Colon
- Gastric
- Pancreatic

Assessment of Ascites

Symptoms Associated with Ascites

Patients report abdominal bloating and pain. Initially, patients describe a feeling that they need larger-waisted clothing and notice an increase in belt size or weight. They may feel nauseated and have a decreased appetite. Some will report increased symptoms of reflux or heartburn. Pronounced ascites can cause dyspnea and orthopnea due to increased pressure on the diaphragm.

Physical Examination

The physical examination may reveal abdominal or inguinal hernia, scrotal edema, and abdominal venous engorgement. Radiological findings show a hazy picture, with distended and separate loops of the bowel. There is a poor definition of the abdominal organs and loss of the psoas muscle shadows. Ultrasound and CT scans may also be used to diagnose ascites.

Management of Ascites

Traditionally, treatment of ascites is palliative because of poor prognosis. Ovarian cancer is one of the few types where the presence of ascites does not necessarily correlate with a poor prognosis. In this case, survival rate can be improved through surgical intervention and adjuvant therapy.

Medical Therapy

Advanced liver disease is associated with central ascites. There is an increase in renal sodium and water retention. Therefore, restricting sodium intake to 100 mmol/day or less along with fluid restriction for patients with moderate to severe hyponatremia (125 mmol/L) may be beneficial. Using potassium-sparing diuretics is also important. Spironolactone (100 to 400 mg/day) is the drug of choice. Furosemide is also helpful at 40 to 80 mg/day to initiate diuresis. Overdiuresis must be avoided. Overdiuresis may precipitate electrolyte imbalance, hepatic encephalopathy, and prerenal failure.

The above regimen of fluid and sodium reduction and diuretics may work for mixed-type ascites, which results from compression of vessels related to tumor and peripheral tumor cells of the parietal or visceral peritoneum as well. Because mixed-type ascites is associated with chylous fluid, adding changes to the diet, such as decreased fat intake and increased medium-chain triglycerides, may be important. Chylous ascites results from tumor infiltration of the retroperitoneal space, causing obstruction of lymphatic flow.

Medium-chain triglyceride oil (Lipisorb) can be used as a calorie source in these patients. Because the lymph system is bypassed, the shorter fatty acid chains are easier to digest.

For patients with refractory ascites and a shortened life expectancy, paracentesis may be the most appropriate therapy. Paracentesis is the most common and effective treatment to relieve ascites. Patients with liver disease can tolerate the removal of up to 5 liters of ascites fluid without an effect on renal function or plasma volume.[12] Although this procedure gives temporary relief of symptoms like the treatment of MBO, palliative care decisions should be based on the goals of care and patients' quality of life. New advances in paracentesis treatment options have improved long-term use to minimize the need for frequent trips to the hospital for the procedure and repeated painful needle sticks.

Paracentesis Catheters

Peritoneovenous shunts (PVS) (Denver or LeVeen shunt) are helpful for the removal of ascites in 75% to 85% of patients. These shunts are used primarily for nonmalignant ascites. The shunt removes fluid from the site, and the fluid is shunted up into the internal jugular vein.

This type of shunt has the advantage of avoiding an external drainage device and can be placed with minimal invasive techniques under conscious sedation. The disadvantages are that they have a high rate of failure related to occlusion and have been associated with pulmonary edema, thrombosis of major veins, seroma formation, leaks, and disseminated intravascular coagulation (DIC).

Pigtail Catheter

Pigtail drainage catheters are used for percutaneous drainage of ascites as well as relief of pleural effusions, abcesses, and biliary tract and renal drainage. They are placed under ultrasound or fluoroscopic guidance as an outpatient procedure and can be intermittently drained to gravity or vacuum bottles. Patients or their family members are taught to manage drainage at home.

Dialysis Catheters

Silastic peritoneal dialysis catheters are providing effective management of malignant ascites. They also can be managed at home easily and can be on gravity drainage or vacuum bottle drainage as needed.

Pleurex Catheter (Denver Biomedical, Denver, Colorado)

This is a single-cuff tunneled Silastic catheter approved for the drainage of malignant plural effusions and malignant ascites. It offers a one-way valve instead of a clamp and can be managed in the home as well.

The management of all of these types of catheters requires careful handling and techniques to prevent infections. Peritonitis, cellulitis, and catheter occlusion are risks.

Nursing Management

Ascites management involves initially understanding the mechanism, then using interventions appropriately. Nurses should employ good supportive care, including skin care to prevent breakdown, and comfort interventions, such as pillow support and loose clothing, whenever possible. Educating the patient and caregivers on the rationale behind fluid and sodium restrictions, when necessary, can help their understanding and compliance. Careful explanation about use of drainage catheters is crucial. Support of the patient and family is crucial throughout the course of illness.

Summary

Managing GI symptoms such as constipation, diarrhea, MBO, and ascites requires thorough assessment skills and knowledge of appropriate pharmacological and nonpharmacological interventions. Excellent symptom management is essential to promote the patient's comfort and dignity.

References

1. Clark K, Currow DC. Assessing constipation in palliative care within a gastroenterology framework. Palliat Med. 2012;26(6):834–841.

2. Twycross R, Sykes N, Mihalyo M, Wilcock A. Stimulant laxatives and opioid-induced constipation. J Pain Symptom Manage. 2012;43(2):306–313.

3. McMillan SC, Tofthagen C, Small B, Karver S, Craig D. Trajectory of medication-induced constipation in patients with cancer. Oncol Nurs Forum. 2013;40(3):E92–E100.

4. Librach SL, Bouvette M, De Angelis C, et al. Consensus recommendations for the management of constipation in patients with advanced, progressive illness. J Pain Symptom Manage. 2010;40:761–773.

5. McMillan SC, Williams FA. Validity and reliability of the Constipation Assessment Scale. Cancer Nurs. 1989;12(3):183–188.

6. Jones C, Goodman M, Drake R, Tookman A. Laxatives or methylnaltrexone for the management of constipation in palliative care patients (Review). Cochrane Database Syst Rev. 2011(8).

7. Weihofen DL, Marino, C. Cancer Survival Cookbook. Los Angeles: Wiley; 1998.

8. Muehlbauer PM, Thorpe D, Davis A, Drabot R, Rawlings BL, Kiker E. Putting evidence into practice: evidence-based interventions to prevent, manage, and treat chemotherapy- and radiotherapy-induced diarrhea. Clin J Oncol Nurs. 2009;13:336–341.

9. Ripamonti CI. Malignant bowel obstruction: tailoring treatment to individual patients. J Support Oncol. 2008;6(3):114–115.

10. Mercadante S, Porzio G. Octreotide for malignant bowel obstruction: twenty years after. Crit Rev Oncol Hematol. 2012;83:388–392.

11. Rath KS, Loseth D, Muscarella P, et al. Outcomes following percutaneous upper gastrointestinal decompressive tube placement for malignant bowel obstruction in ovarian cancer. Gynecol Oncol. 2013;129:103–106.

12. Becker G, Galandi D, Blum HE. Malignant ascites: systematic review and guideline for treatment. Eur J Cancer. 2006;42:589–597.

Appendix

Patient Care: Pain Management Test Questions and Answers

1. Tingling, burning, and electrical sensation are common descriptors of which of the following types of pain?
   a. bone
   b. visceral
   c. neuropathic
   d. psychogenic

2. Which of the following is MOST commonly associated with uncontrolled chronic pain?
   a. grimacing
   b. agitation
   c. depression
   d. hallucinations

3. Bone metastasis should be suspected when a patient describes leg pain as
   a. sharp, stabbing, and decreases with movement.
   b. aching, throbbing, and worse with movement.
   c. burning, localized, and not affected by movement.
   d. cramping, generalized, and relieved with movement.

4. A patient calls stating that he has new pain in his right hip. He describes the pain as being sharp and radiating to his buttock. When he moves, he feels pain in the inner aspect of his right knee. The nurse should FIRST
   a. arrange for further patient evaluation.
   b. notify the physician of a new hip fracture.
   c. instruct the patient to be up with assistance only.
   d. recommend the patient take ibuprofen 400 mg PO every 6 hours.

5. A behavioral pain scale is appropriate to use
   a. when a patient refuses to rate the pain.
   b. when a patient does not speak English.
   c. when a patient has significant cognitive impairment.
   d. to validate a patient's pain rating.

6. Somatic pain caused by a tumor pressing on soft tissue is MOST likely described as
   a. aching.
   b. burning.
   c. squeezing.
   d. cramping.

7. A patient with head and neck cancer complains of dull aching pain over the left jaw with intermittent, sharp, shooting pain over the left cheek. Which of the following types of pain is being exhibited?
   a. somatic and neuropathic
   b. central and peripheral
   c. visceral and musculoskeletal
   d. cutaneous and nociceptive

8. Which of the following would be the MOST appropriate adjuvant medicine for treating bone pain?
   a. acetaminophen
   b. antianxiety agents
   c. muscle relaxants
   d. nonsteroidal antiinflammatory drugs

9. When initiating around-the-clock opioids, the nurse should instruct the patient and family that the sedative effect usually lasts
   a. a few days.
   b. a few weeks.
   c. several hours.
   d. throughout the course of treatment.

10. Which of the following adjuvants to opioids is MOST often added to the pain regimen for controlling nerve pain?
    a. adrenergics
    b. antispasmodics
    c. antidepressants
    d. antiinflammatories

11. An important role of antineoplastic drugs in palliative care is to
    a. maintain hope for remission.
    b. promote improved immune responses.
    c. decrease side effects of treatments.
    d. reduce tumor mass to relieve symptoms.

12. Which of the following is the MOST common conversion ratio for changing from oral to parenteral morphine?
    a. 1:1
    b. 3:1
    c. 4:1
    d. 6:1

13. When using an opioid as an epidural analgesia, lethargy and constipation will occur how often?
    a. as frequently as in oral administration
    b. less frequently than with oral administration
    c. more frequently than with oral administration
    d. as frequently as in intravenous administration

14. Which of the following bowel management protocols is essential when a patient starts a regimen of opioid analgesia?
    a. high-fiber diet
    b. milk of magnesia 30 ml twice a day
    c. stool softener with a stimulant every day
    d. Fleet enema every 3 days if no bowel movement occurs

15. Which of the following topical agents is MOST appropriate in treating superficial neuropathic pain?
    a. lidocaine patch
    b. hydrocortisone gel
    c. ketoconazole cream
    d. diphenhydramine lotion

16. The appropriateness of massage therapy for pain treatment depends primarily on
    a. the patient's age.
    b. absence of lung disease.
    c. absence of bone metastases.
    d. the patient's personal preferences.

17. Which of the following is a potential side effect of opioid use?
    a. diarrhea
    b. azotemia
    c. hematuria
    d. urinary retention

18. A patient who is terminally ill experiences nausea and vomiting only with movement. Which of the following medications would be MOST effective?
    a. meclizine
    b. lorazepam
    c. haloperidol
    d. metoclopramide

Answers

1. c. neuropathic
2. c. depression
3. b. aching, throbbing, and worse with movement
4. a. arrange for further patient evaluation
5. c. when a patient has significant cognitive impairment
6. a. aching
7. a. somatic and neuropathic
8. d. nonsteroidal antiinflammatory drugs
9. a. a few days.
10. c. antidepressants
11. d. reduce tumor mass to relieve symptoms
12. b. 3:1
13. b. less frequently than with oral administration
14. c. stool softener with a stimulant every day
15. a. lidocaine patch
16. d. the patient's personal preferences.
17. d. urinary retention
18. a. meclizine

Index

143